Carcinogenicity Testing

Carcinogenicity Testing: Principles and Problems

Proceedings of a Symposium held at the Royal College of Physicians, London, on Friday, December 2, 1977

Edited by
A. D. Dayan

The Wellcome Research Laboratories, Beckenham, Kent,

and

R. W. Brimblecombe

Smith, Kline and French Laboratories, Welwyn Garden City, Herts.

University Park Press
Baltimore

Published in the USA and Canada by

University Park Press
233 East Redwood Street
Baltimore, Maryland 21202

Published in the UK by

MTP Press Ltd
St Leonard's House
St Leonardgate
Lancaster
England

Library of Congress Catalog Card Number 78–56957

ISBN 0–8391–1283–1

Printed in Great Britain

Contents

List of Contributors vii

Preface ix

1 Long-term tests for carcinogenicity – the pathologist's view *R. L. Carter* 1
Commentary 16

2 The predictive value or otherwise of conventional carcinogenicity studies
D. E. Stevenson, E. Thorpe and P. F. Hunt 19
Commentary 27

3 The predictive value of biochemical tests for carcinogenicity
J. Bridges and J. R. Fry 29
Commentary 53

4 The predictive value of microbiological tests for carcinogenicity
M. H. L. Green 55
Commentary 62

5 Biochemical mechanisms of carcinogenicity
T. A. Connors 65
Commentary 77

6 The economics of carcinogenicity testing
D. M. Conning 79
Commentary 87

7 Lifetime carcinogenic studies in rodents viewed from the standpoint of experimental design – weaknesses and alternatives
D. Salsburg 89
Commentary 103

8 Problems facing the regulatory authorities. I: Problems involved with medicinal products
G. Jones 105

9 Problems facing the regulatory authorities. II: Problems in interpreting and implementing results from carcinogenicity studies
E. M. B. Smith 113
Commentary 117

10 The tetrazolium test for skin carcinogenicity
O. H. Iversen 119

Index 125

List of Contributors

J. Bridges
Department of Biochemistry, University of Surrey, Guildford, Surrey.

R. L. Carter
Haddow Laboratories, Institute of Cancer Research and the Royal Marsden Hospital, Sutton, Surrey.

D. M. Conning
ICI Central Toxicology Laboratory, Macclesfield, Cheshire.

T. A. Connors
MRC Toxicology Unit, Carshalton, Surrey.

J. R. Fry
Department of Biochemistry, University of Surrey, Guildford, Surrey.

M. H. L. Green
MRC Cell Mutation Unit, University of Sussex, Falmer, Brighton.

P. F. Hunt
Shell Toxicology Laboratory, Sittingbourne Research Centre, Sittingbourne, Kent.

O. H. Iversen
Institute of Pathology, University of Oslo, Norway.

G. Jones

Medicines Division, Department of Health and Social Security, London.

D. Salsburg

Department of Clinical Research, Pfizer Central Research, Groton, Connecticut, USA.

E. M. B. Smith

Department of Health and Social Security, London.

D. E. Stevenson

Shell Toxicology Laboratory, Sittingbourne Research Centre, Sittingbourne, Kent.

E. Thorpe

Shell Toxicology Laboratory, Sittingbourne Research Centre, Sittingbourne, Kent.

Preface

To test a candidate drug or other chemical substance for carcinogenic activity may well be the most difficult challenge faced by a toxicologist. A compound so far in development will already have cost several man-years and many million pounds, and then the expert is asked to devise an apparently quite simple test which will answer definitively and with considerable sensitivity whether the material will produce neoplasms in two species, and from that to suggest the likely hazard to other far-removed species, probably man and possibly domesticated animals. On his results and their interpretation depend all the effort and resources so far expended, the considerable cost of the carcinogenicity test itself, and the enormous burden if not of proof at least of prediction of *safety*, which will lead to the huge expense of industrial development and studies in man, or of *carcinogenicity*, which will inevitably result in expensive abandonment of the project, or of its curtailment. The human and economic reliance on carcinogenicity testing is almost total, and yet how often is an analysis made of the theoretical basis of such tests, of the biochemical and pathological implications of current practice, of their statistical power, and of their cost-effectiveness?

This book is an edited account of a short symposium organized in London in December 1977. The speakers have provided accounts of their contributions, some before and others after the meeting. The audience was chosen to represent university and other academic interests, British regulatory bodies, and the pharmaceutical, chemical and agro-chemical industries. Their discussions with the speakers were recorded and the account given here has been edited for brevity whilst attempting to preserve the thrust of the arguments.

The contributed talks and the questions covered most aspects of the practice of carcinogenicity testing and its effects on industrial development and economics. There was particular emphasis on the problems of experimental design, of pathological interpretation and statistical analysis of the findings and on the biochemical and other biological factors that may make it impossible to transfer results from one species to another. Short-term tests of mutagenicity were appraised with enthusiasm mingled with the caution appropriate to any novel and fashionable but as yet inadequately proven techniques. Finally, the attitudes of the British Committee on the Safety of Medicines and the Department of Health and Social Security were described in an account of the official view on which materials should be tested and how and when.

There was relatively little discussion of what should be done with the information obtained from such expensive and therefore virtually unrepeatable experiments. If the results are negative, i.e. there is not an excess of tumours in treated animals, then the compound will generally be accepted as non-carcinogenic – at least under those experimental circumstances. However, should the substance appear to produce neoplasms, then there will be concern with whether it might have acted directly or after metabolic activation, via an indirect effect on the endocrine glands or whether the effect is due to contaminants in the diet, and whether the biological and biochemical mechanisms and responses might be unique to the species involved.

Perhaps the deepest and least well understood points and therefore ones that were barely touched upon, were how to use our scanty knowledge of mechanism in carcinogenicity as a guide through the molecular maze of synthetic chemistry, and how best to use results from relatively small numbers of rodents to predict hazard for man. On several occasions more or less hypothetical assumptions have been made about the shape and slope of the dose/response curve in animals to diverse carcinogens and the results used to calculate the degree of risk to human populations. With as much scientific freedom 'safety margins' have been assumed in an entirely arbitrary fashion and different degrees of risk have been computed. No one yet can decide what is correct, but information is being obtained that will help to clarify mechanisms of carcinogenicity and to delineate the hazard to man. At present considerable care is taken to avoid exposure of the population to new or old carcinogens, and if such a risk is taken, it is only under extreme conditions sharply delineated by past experiences. In some ways the problem of assessment of safety and hence of risk and benefit of chemicals is like that of radiation about 30 years ago; methods are still primitive, knowledge is scanty and estimates of hazard can only be far from accurate.

The impression given must be one of uncertainty, as was often demonstrated at this symposium. However, although empirical in the extreme, present day methods of testing and interpretation have had demonstrable successes. We must await better knowledge of the mechanisms and actions of carcinogenic chemicals before a rigidly scientific balance can be drawn between the value of a compound and the potential or actual hazards of its use.

The Editors are grateful to their colleagues for their persistent enthusiasm and unfailing help, especially to Dr D. A. Stevenson (B.A.A.), Miss D. Wilson and Mr R. Summers (Wellcome Foundation), Dr S. F. Sullman and Miss E. Donnelly (A.B.P.I.). They wish also to thank Mrs J. Fagleson, Mr M. Lister and the publishers for their speedy and flexible co-operation.

A. D. Dayan
R. W. Brimblecombe

London, April 1978

1

Long-term tests for carcinogenicity: the pathologist's view

R. L. Carter

INTRODUCTION

This chapter deals in a selective fashion with two topics. Certain general aspects of long-term carcinogenicity tests are briefly described. This provides a context for the main section which discusses some of the qualitative problems in characterizing and evaluating induced neoplasms, particularly in terms of their predictive relevance for man.

GENERAL ASPECTS OF LONG-TERM CARCINOGENICITY TESTS

These may be summarized under three main headings: the test compound, the test animal and the test procedure. Each comprises important and often controversial matters and, for a full account, the reader is referred to References 1–7 at the end of this chapter, and to other parts of this book.

The test compound

The main considerations here are the need to test the active ingredient or the formulated product, the physical and chemical properties of the material, and the presence of impurities. Particular solvents may give rise to toxic effects, but these tend to be more frequently associated with acute and subacute consequences involving, in particular, the eye and the skin. Information relating to pharmacokinetics, intermediate metabolism and degradation, and tissue residues is particularly important. Knowledge of the patterns of metabolic transformation, and of the anatomical locations where such changes occur, may be invaluable when the wider hazards of a potential tumour-inducing substance have to be evaluated (see p. 12).

The test animal

This involves the selection of appropriate species and strains, with optimal numbers at an optimal age maintained under optimal conditions. Two species of rodents are currently advocated, and most schedules recommend the use of outbred animals from a closed colony with well characterized patterns of background neoplastic and non-neoplastic disease (see p. 3). Details of animal husbandry and diet are important in that they have a direct bearing (through survival) on the duration of the test; also because dietary factors affect the yield of tumours. This is an important topic with obvious practical implications which merits more detailed consideration.

Diet

That dietary factors may affect tumour development was recognized in the 1930s when it was shown that riboflavin inhibited tumour induction in rats fed 4-dimethylaminoazobenzene. Detailed studies by Tannenbaum and Silverstone [8] (see also Clayson [9]) showed that dietary restriction, or restriction of caloric intake, resulted in a decreased incidence of various tumour types in several strains of rats and mice. The subject has been re-examined by Roe and Tucker [10] and some of their results in overfed, affluent mice are summarized in Table 1.1.

Three points are raised here. First, the reason for the increased tumour

Table 1.1 Cancers in affluent mice

Feeding	*Total tumours at 18 months*	*Tumours*			
		lung	*liver*	*lymphoma*	*other*
4 g diet per day; one mouse per cage	4	1	1	2	0
5 g diet per day; one mouse per cage	4	2	0	1	1
Diet *ad libitum;* one mouse per cage	32	15	2	11	4
Diet *ad libitum;* five mice per cage	23	8	6	9	0

Forty male Swiss mice per group; standard pellet diet; similar survival in all groups. Data from Roe and Tucker[10].

incidence in mice fed *ad libitum* is not clear. Some animal diets may be variably contaminated by known carcinogens, such as aflatoxin and the nitrosamines. Other chemical contaminants, notably the organochlorine pesticides, can act as powerful microsomal inducing agents (Depending on the prevailing conditions, such inducers can either enhance or inhibit chemical carcinogenesis.) Secondly, should the experimenter aim for standard *composition* of his diets (which usually means the use of semi-synthetic and highly expensive feeds) or for standard *consumption*? Thirdly, there is the question of extrapolation to man, particularly to overfed man in industrialized societies. The contributory role of dietary factors in certain human cancers (oesophagus, stomach, large intestine, liver) is attracting increased attention (Doll [11]).

Background incidence of disease

It is difficult to overemphasize the importance of continuous monitoring of animal colonies for the incidence of 'spontaneous' tumours and major non-neoplastic lesions in control animals. The incidence of certain common spontaneous neoplasms in rodents – arising in breast, lung, liver, lymphoid system, the endocrine glands – often fluctuates widely, and it is essential to know the range of incidence of such tumours. (It is equally important to know *why* such fluctuations occur, but information is rarely available: factors within the colony such as a change in the gene pool, a virus infection or a new chemical, inadvertently introduced, almost always remain speculative.)

The test procedure

The principal topics here are the route of administration of the test compound, the dose-levels and the duration of the test.

The route of administration is determined by the eventual use or exposure of the proposed compound. The respiratory tract is an important target for chemicals used in industry, and improved methods for chronic inhalation toxicology are needed.

There is now a tendency, with improved animal husbandry, for carcinogenicity tests to be extended beyond the hitherto conventional time limits of 18 months for mice and 24 months for rats; some protocols advocate termination at the point where 20% of the control group are still alive. This approach can be criticized on the grounds that the background level of some spontaneous tumours may become so high as to vitiate the entire test. Certainly the range and variety of spontaneous neoplasms is frequently increased, but this makes for a more realistic test situation. The possible physiological and biochemical consequences of ageing on tumour development, in the course of a life-span test, are ill-understood. Such changes include age-related structural and functional alterations in the target site(s) and in the main metabolizing parenchymal organs, alterations in endocrine function, and alterations in immune function. Whether such changes impinge on tumour development in any way, particularly during the later stages, is not known, but the subject deserves attention.

There is scope for discussion on the question of *interim killing* of animals. Given the ever-increasing costs of long-term tests, it is essential that each one yields the maximum amount of information. There are grounds for regarding them as tests for chronic toxicity rather than as tests exclusively for carcinogenicity. If, therefore, certain changes are noted in a previous subacute (90-day) toxicity test, it may be prudent to pursue these abnormalities in the subsequent chronic test and include extra animals for interim killings.

The autopsy and subsequent microscopy

There are four absolute requirements to bear in mind.

(a) high autopsy rate;
(b) sustained technical competence in dissecting, observing and recording;
(c) all macroscopic findings to be available for correlation with microscopy;
(d) prompt recognition of 'special circumstances'.

Most of these points are self-evident. A high autopsy rate presupposes close, regular surveillance of all animals on test. Sick animals must be killed and, whenever possible, the reasons for their deterioration determined. Standard records are essential and the need to be alert for 'special circumstances' should be stressed. If, for example, macroscopic liver nodules are found it is essential that the tissues are minutely examined, at autopsy and during subsequent microscopy, for metastases. Again, the presence of bladder lesions should alert the operator to check carefully for calculi.

In reporting histological findings it is essential that standard nomenclature is used whenever possible. It should, however, be borne in mind that such nomenclature has almost always been formulated for human lesions. Most of the time it can be applied to lesions in experimental animals quite adequately, but there are situations where human-derived terminology proves inadequate (see p. 8). For tumours, each neoplasm is classified and the eventual yield of benign and malignant neoplasms, for each test and control group, is summarized in a part-quantitative and part-qualitative form. It is with certain qualitative aspects of experimental tumours that the rest of this chapter is concerned. Quantitative aspects of carcinogenesis testing are discussed in Chapter 2.

QUALITATIVE APPRAISAL OF TUMOURS IN CARCINOGENICITY TESTS

What might be regarded as a reasonably straightforward set of results is shown in Table 1.2. Two situations are illustrated – (1) tumours of a given

Table 1.2 Two patterns of results in carcinogenicity tests

Tumours of one or more type
(1) Seen in test animals only
(2) Seen in test and control animals
In test groups:
More tumours
Earlier occurrence
More tumours per animal
Dose–response seen in (1) and (2).

type develop solely in the test groups, showing a clear dose–response relationship; and (2) a particular tumour type is found both in the test and control groups but, in the test groups, the tumours are more numerous, occur earlier and again show a dose–response relationship. Situations (1) and (2) may co-exist. Given the formidable problems of interpretation which some carcinogenicity tests present (see later sections), it is worth noting that a sizeable proportion of positive tests produce reasonably clear-cut results along the lines illustrated by Table 1.2. Not that the illustrations shown in this table are wholly straightforward: it is not clear, for example, whether the induction of an uncommon tumour type and the increased incidence (in the test groups) of a tumour occurring at lower incidence in untreated controls necessarily reflects the same mechanism. There is, however, no positive evidence that two different mechanisms are operating in these circumstances.

Some results from carcinogenicity tests are much more problematic. 'Debatable lesions' are, of course, no more common in laboratory animals than in man; but the experimental situation, exemplified in the long-term carcinogenicity test, carries particularly wide and far-reaching implications. Some of the general difficulties presented are shown in Table 1.3. They are illustrated here with reference to neoplastic lesions in three target organs: lungs, breast and liver.

Tumours of the lungs

The histopathological patterns of the main malignant tumours found in man and in laboratory rodents are summarized in Table 1.4. The *rat*, in which spontaneous pulmonary tumours are rare, shows a variety of morphological patterns which correspond quite closely to human lesions. The small cell anaplastic ('oat-cell') carcinoma is the main exception, as it is questionable whether this tumour has been induced experimentally.

Pulmonary neoplasms in *mice* are more difficult to evaluate. These multifocal aveolar cell lesions occur spontaneously at a high incidence in some strains (A, SWR), and both spontaneous and induced lesions show a wide spectrum

Table 1.3 Some dilemmas in carcinogenicity tests for the pathologist

1. Development of experimental tumours is often an evolving process, observed at several phases.
2. Orthodox descriptive pathology may be inadequate.
3. Terminology – 'a mixture of descriptive, evaluative and predictive meanings' (Smithers [36]) – may be imprecise and controversial.
4. Background levels of 'spontaneous' tumours and related lesions fluctuate in untreated control animals.
5. Tumours in animals often differ from corresponding tumours in man.
6. Licensing and statutory bodies require unequivocal conclusions; nomenclature may thus carry ultimate economic, legal and political connotations*.

* See, for example, Refs. 37 and 38.

of morphological appearances (Table 1.5). Resemblance to the rare alveolar cell carcinomas of man, which are almost certainly variants of adenocarcinomas, is tenuous. The two ends of the spectrum in Table 1.5 – focal hyperplasia and invasive metastasising carcinoma – are easy enough to recognize, but the demarcation of diagnostic categories within the spectrum becomes

Table 1.4 Lung carcinomas in man and rodents

Man		*Rodents*
	Squamous cell carcinoma*	
	Adenocarcinoma	
		Mucoepidermoid carcinoma
Anaplastic 'oat cell' carcinoma†		
		Alveolar cell carcinoma‡
	Different patterns of invasion and metastasis	

* Rare in mice.
† ? ever produced experimentally.
‡ Rare in rats.
Details from References 22, 39–41

increasingly difficult. Purely morphological criteria are highly subjective (here as in many similar contexts), and most other means of investigation – electron microscopy, biochemistry, immunology, tumour markers – have not been pursued in any detail.

Table 1.5 Alveolar cell neoplasms in mice

Within lungs	Alveolar cell (type II) hyperplasia Adenoma Carcinoma (glandular, cystic, papillary, solid)
Outside lungs	Carcinoma, undifferentiated 'Carcinosarcoma' Sarcoma

Details from References 22, 40, 42, 43.

Tumours of the breast

Although breast cancers are common in man and in rodents their pathology differs in many respects (Table 1.6). The only morphological overlap is seen with respect to well-differentiated carcinomas which are rare in women but predominate in rodents. Most mammary cancers in rats and mice are multiple, have little stroma and show a high degree of hormone-sensitivity. Their metastatic capacity is small. The background incidence of mammary tumours in several strains of untreated female rats (Sprague-Dawley, Fischer) and mice (C3H, DBA, A) is high, and the development of multiple, often rapidly

Table 1.6 Breast carcinomas in man and rodents

Man	*Rodents*
Scirrhous Medullary Colloid — 90%	
Comedocarcinoma	Comedocarcinoma
Papillary carcinoma	Papillary carcinoma
Tubular carcinoma	Tubular carcinoma
Different patterns of invasion and metastasis	Different patterns of invasion and metastasis

Details from References 22, 40, 42, 44, 45.

growing tumours may lead to the premature end of an experiment. The aetiological factors involved in the rat and mouse differ, particularly with respect to the implication of mammary tumour viruses; and the antecedent hyperplastic alevolar nodules found in mice do not appear to have any counterpart in the rat.

Much attention has been paid recently to mammary lesions in *dogs* used for long-term testing of proposed oral contraceptives [12]. Quite apart from the changes involved in moving to a less familiar, long-lived species of test animal, these drug-induced changes in the breast pose considerable problems in diagnosis. Morphological appearances differ profoundly from those seen in man or laboratory rodents [13]. The canine mixed tumours, in particular, have no counterpart in other familiar species; these are special tumours which require special expertise for their appraisal. The critical role of diagnostic histopathology here is emphasized in Table 1.7 which illustrates the variety of morphological findings in 60 nodules excised from beagles after 4 years treatment with two progestogens.

Table 1.7 Mammary nodules in progestogen-treated beagles; 4 years

	Control	*Megestrol**	*Chlormadinone†*
Nodular hyperplasia	0	27	12
Benign mixed tumour	0	5	4
Adenocarcinoma	0	0	1
Duct ectasia	0	3	0
Fat necrosis	0	1	0
Other	0	2	5

* Megestrol. Combined data from three groups fed 0·01, 0·1 and 0·25 mg/day.
† Chlormadinone. One dose level: 0·25 mg/day.
Details from Reference 46.

Tumours of the liver

The histopathology of *overtly malignant* liver carcinomas in rats and mice, showing local invasion and distant metastases, tallies quite closely with the corresponding human tumours (see Table 1.8). Hepatocellular carcinomas, often multifocal, predominate. They show a spectrum of morphological patterns which, in rodents, bears no relation to the aetiological agent. The incidence of cholangiocellular carcinomas in rodents is low though cholangiofibromas are more common (in rats) and ductular cell proliferation is a frequent early response to liver carcinogens both in rats and mice. In contrast to tumours of the lungs and breast, the pattern of spread of hepatocellular carcinomas in rodents is similar to that found in man, with local infiltration within the liver substance, spread to the portal vein, and metastases in lungs and porta hepatis and coeliac lymph nodes.

It is, however, the non-invasive, non-metastasizing, proliferative liver lesions which present particular problems in terminology, classification and evaluation.

Table 1.8 Liver carcinomas in man and rodents

<table>
<tr><th>Man</th><th>Rodents</th></tr>
<tr><td colspan="2">(A) Hepatocellular carcinoma</td></tr>
<tr><td colspan="2">Trabecular</td></tr>
<tr><td colspan="2">Adenoid</td></tr>
<tr><td colspan="2">Anaplastic</td></tr>
<tr><td colspan="2">('hepatoblastoma')</td></tr>
<tr><td colspan="2">(B) Cholangiocellular carcinoma*</td></tr>
<tr><td colspan="2">Mucus-secreting</td></tr>
<tr><td colspan="2">Papillary</td></tr>
<tr><td colspan="2">Broadly similar patterns of intra- and extra- hepatic spread</td></tr>
</table>

* Incidence disputed in rodents. Main evidence rests on the presence of basement membranes in the electron microscope, and of PAS-positive mucins.

Details from References 18, 22, 40, 47–50.

Rats

It is generally agreed that hyperplastic foci of liver cells – called 'nodules' in this account – represent an important stage in the development of hepatocellular carcinoma. Most if not all hepatocarcinogens give rise to nodules, with or without an accompanying cirrhosis. Isotopically labelled hepatocarcinogens, such as 2-acetylaminofluorene (2-AAF), have been localized within the nodules. The early morphological changes of malignancy – in the form of islands of pleomorphic and hyperbasophilic cells – arise within the nodules. Similar focal lesions are thought to provide the origin for the multicentric hepatocellular carcinomas which develop in the cirrhotic liver of man. However, any simple correlation between nodules and carcinomas breaks down for various reasons. Hepatocarcinogens commonly evoke numerous focal nodules, but most of them are initially capable of 'remodelling or differentiating', to use Farber's term (see Refs. 14–16). Depending on the experimental conditions, a smaller number of these nodules lose their capacity to regress; and a still smaller proportion will eventually develop the 'islands of malignancy' (Farber [15]) which represent early carcinoma. Liver carcinogenesis is thus seen as a reductive, highly selective, evolving series of events, a crude summary of which is given in Table 1.9. The practical problems stem from the fact that it is impossible to distinguish between nodules which can 'remodel and differentiate', and those which cannot, up to the stage when the latter begin to develop histological changes of focal malignancy. Until this point is reached, morphology, electron microscopy, histochemistry, biochemistry, immunology, transplantation studies and karyotype analyses have failed to show up any differences between them. The α-fetoprotein marker has proved unreliable but recent studies with a new marker – the pre-neoplastic or PN antigen – may lead to some advances.

Table 1.9 Pathogenesis of hepatocellular carcinoma in rats (Farber)

1. Entire liver provides the target organ. Ultrastructural changes in liver cells and ductular cells.*
2. Focal liver cell proliferation: EARLY NODULES,† capable of 'differentiation and remodelling'
3. Focal liver cell proliferation: LATE NODULES,† incapable of 'differentiation and remodelling'.
4. HEPATOCELLULAR carcinomas.

↓ A REDUCTIVE, SELECTIVE SERIES OF EVENTS

* ? Regional variation within the liver lobule, in 'acinoperipheral' and 'acinocentral' regions [51].

† For a possible exception to the general association between potential hepatocarcinogens and the development of nodules which eventually become persistent and irreversible, see Reference 53.

Details from References 14–16, 52, 54.

There are several other problems to note. With some carcinogens the balance between inducing predominantly reversible and predominantly irreversible nodules is a fine one: three 3-week feeding cycles with 2-AAF gave rise to regressing liver nodules, but a fourth cycle induced irreversible nodules and hepatocellular carcinomas. Is morphological regression of 'early' nodules a truly complete and permanent process? To what extent are the nodules, at any stage, functionally heterogeneous according to criteria which have not yet been recognized? And at what stage does the pre-neoplastic cell population appear?

Mice

The situation with regard to non-invasive proliferative lesions in the mouse verges on the chaotic. Unlike the rat, spontaneous liver lesions are common, especially in males of certain strains (CBA, C3H). The incidence of both spontaneous and induced lesions is particularly susceptible to modulating factors in addition to strain and sex. These include age, diet (see p. 2), stress, endocrine status, exogenous chemicals and viruses [17]. Morphological criteria demarcating hyperplastic nodules and non-invasive neoplasms are controversial [18] and it is still disputed whether transplantability of lesions bears any relation to histology [19–22]. Indeed, the interpretation of transplantability *per se* is controversial: is it a specific measure of malignancy or, more generally, of neoplasia? The need still remains for more detailed studies of the development of liver nodules and neoplasms, spontaneous or induced, tracing their evolution by morphology (including electron microscopy and histochemistry) supplemented by biochemistry, immunology, virology, and marker substances.

Most pressing of all is the practical problem in evaluating compounds, some of them of considerable value and importance, which evoke an increased incidence of proliferative liver lesions in mice *as an isolated finding* – that is, unaccompanied by any increased incidence of tumours at other sites, or any tumours in any other test species [23]. Such compounds include chlorinated hydrocarbons, especially some of the organochlorine pesticides, phenobarbitone and griseofulvin [21,24–28]. In the case of the organochlorine pesticides, most of the lesions fall into the disputed hyperplasia – non-invasive neoplasm category, but there is certainly a small proportion (~5%) of metastasizing hepatocellular carcinomas. Dose–response relationships have been noted in several experiments and positive results obtained in different strains of mice [26,28]. The evaluation of such results is enormously contentious; and even the most superficial analysis of the various conclusions that have been reached would fill another chapter. The induction of these liver lesions in mice, alone, cannot be ignored when attempting to extrapolate potential carcinogenic risks to man; the pragmatic view is that they should be regarded as potential danger signals indicating the need for further investigations. These include studies of mechanisms in the mouse and studies in another test species. Studies with human liver microsomes may be valuable when considering possible homologous pathways of metabolic activation (cf. p. 12). Metabolic mechanisms specific to the mouse have been described in relation to griseofulvin, involving porphyrins [24,27], and evidence is accumulating for species specificity in relation to dieldrin and to phenobarbitone [29]. Far more important is the contribution from *human epidemiology*, in the case of compounds which have already been in use for sufficiently long periods of time. The strongest evidence that a substance is carcinogenic for man is epidemiological, and suitable chronically exposed populations provide invaluable information. Examples include workers concerned with the manufacture and formulation of some organochlorine pesticides [30–32] and epileptics on maintenance phenobarbitone [33]. Risk–benefit analyses will also have to be considered.

Man

A final comment may be made to correct any impression that the interpretative problems posed by liver nodules are peculiar to rats and mice. 'Debatable', non-malignant liver nodules are being described with increasing frequency, particularly in women, where there may be an association with the

Table 1.10 Some non-malignant 'liver nodules' in man

Liver cell adenoma
Adenomatous hyperplasia
Focal nodular hyperplasia
Hamartoma

Details from References 55, 56.

use of oral contraceptives – Table 1.10. There are at least eleven synonyms for this group of conditions [34]; and their pathogenesis and natural history are both obscure.

CONCLUSIONS

Experience in the last 20–30 years suggests that the conventional long-term carcinogenicity test provides a reasonably adequate model for detecting strong chemical carcinogens. In general, a standard assay can be expected to show a rise in the development of compound-associated tumours of the order of ~3% or greater. Clearly a risk factor of this magnitude is wholly unacceptable in human terms, and it must be admitted that there is no suitable animal model for testing weak carcinogens*. Even for strong carcinogens, the standard assay is oversimplified and several details of design still need to be modified.

Three more general needs should also be noted:

1. To clarify the biochemical mode(s) of action of putative carcinogens with particular respect to species variation and homology with man.
2. To clarify the development and pathogenesis of the neoplastic and hyperplastic lesions, both spontaneous and those associated with test compounds. The newer, more functionally orientated, approaches of biochemistry, immunology and marker substances need to be more fully deployed.

* We are profoundly ignorant of the consequences of exposure to low concentrations of weak carcinogens, particularly over a long period of time (cf. Barnes [35]). How much damage is inflicted on the target macromolecules? How much of this damage can be repaired *in vivo*? And even if an irreversible sequence of events is set in train, what is the relation between concentration of carcinogen and the latent period before tumours appear? These seemingly theoretical considerations have immediate practical relevance when it comes to deciding on the validity (or otherwise) of setting threshold values for exposure.

3. To collate more closely the experimental and epidemiological aspects. The results of carcinogenicity testing must be set alongside the results of epidemiology whenever possible.

The consolidation and diversification of information which is advocated here forms part of a very simple and practical objective: the more effective protection of people.

References

1 WHO Technical Report Series (1969). *Principles for the Testing and Evaluation of Drugs for Carcinogenicity*. No. 426. (Geneva)

2 WHO Technical Report Series (1974). *Assessment of the Carcinogenicity and Mutagenicity of Chemicals*. No. 546. (Geneva)

3 UICC (1969). *Carcinogenicity Testing*. (Geneva)

4 FDA (1971). Cancer testing in the safety evaluation of food additives and pesticides. *Toxicol. Appl. Pharmacol.*, **20,** 419

5 *Health & Welfare*, Canada (1973). The testing of chemicals for carcinogenicity, mutagenicity and teratogenicity

6 NCI (1976). *Guidelines for Carcinogen Bioassay in Small Rodents*. (Washington: US Department of Health, Education and Welfare)

7 Golberg, L. (ed.) (1974). *Carcinogenesis Testing of Chemicals*. (Cleveland, Ohio: CRC Press, Inc.)

8 Tannenbaum, A. and Silverstone, H. (1957). Nutrition and the genesis of tumours. In R. W. Raven, (ed.) *Cancer*, vol. 1, pp. 308–334. (London: Butterworth)

9 Clayson, D. B. (1975). Nutrition and experimental carcinogenesis: a review. *Cancer Res.*, **35,** 3292

10 Roe, F. J. C. and Tucker, M. J. (1973). Recent developments in the design of carcinogenicity tests on laboratory animals. *Proc. Europ. Soc. Study Drug Toxicity*, **15,** 171

11 Doll, R. (1977). Strategy for detection of cancer hazards to man. *Nature (Lond.)*, **265,** 589

12 Committee on Safety of Medicines (1972). *Carcinogenicity Tests of Oral Contraceptives*. (London: HMSO)

13 Strandberg, J. D. and Goodman, D. G. (1974). Animal models of human disease: canine mammary neoplasia. *Am. J. Pathol.*, **75,** 225

14 Farber, E. (1973). Hyperplastic liver nodules. In H. Busch (ed.). *Methods in Cancer Research*, vol. VII, pp. 345–375. (New York and London: Academic Press)

15 Farber, E. (1976a). On the pathogenesis of experimental hepatocellular carcinoma. In K. Okuda and R. L. Peters (eds.). *Hepatocellular Carcinoma*, pp. 3–22. (New York and London: John Wiley & Sons)

16 Farber, E. (1976b). The pathology of experimental liver cancer. In H. M. Cameron, D. A. Linsell and G. P. Warwick (eds.). *Liver Cell Cancer*, pp. 243–277. (Amsterdam, New York and Oxford: Elsevier)

17 Warwick, G. P. (1971). Metabolism of liver carcinogens and other factors influencing liver cancer induction. In *Liver Cancer*, pp. 121–157. (Lyon: IARC Scientific Publications, No. 1)

18 Butler, W. H. (1971). Pathology of liver cancer in experimental animals. In *Liver Cancer*, pp. 30–41. (Lyon: IARC Scientific Publications No. 1)

19 Andervont, H. B. and Dunn, T. B. (1952). Transplantation of spontaneous and induced hepatomas in inbred mice. *J. Natl. Cancer Inst.*, **13,** 455

20 Reuber, M. D. (1971). Morphological and biologic correlation of hyperplastic and neoplastic hepatic lesions occurring 'spontaneously' in C3H X Y hybrid mice. *Br. J. Cancer,* **25,** 538

21 Thorpe, E. and Walker, A. I. T. (1973). The toxicology of dieldrin (HEOD). II. Comparative long-term oral toxicity studies in mice with dieldrin, DDT, phenobarbitone, γ-BHC and γ-BHC. *Food Cosmet. Toxicol.,* **11,** 433

22 Stewart, H. L. (1975). Comparative aspects of certain cancers, In F. F. Becker (ed.). *Cancer, A Comprehensive Treatise,* vol. 4, pp. 303–374. (New York: Plenum Press)

23 Tomatis, L., Partensky, C. and Montesano, R. (1973). The predictive value of mouse liver tumour induction in carcinogenicity testing – a literature survey. *Int. J. Cancer,* **12,** 1

24 Hurst, E. W. and Paget, G. E. (1963). Protoporphyrin, cirrhosis and hepatomata in the livers of mice given griseofulvin. *Br. J. Dermatol.,* **73,** 105

25 IARC (1972). *IARC Monographs on the Evaluation of Carcinogenic Risk of Chemicals to Man,* Vol. 1. (Lyon)

26 IARC (1974). *IARC Monographs on the Evaluation of Carcinogenic Risk of Chemicals to Man.* Vol. 5: *Some Organochlorine Pesticides.* (Lyon)

27 IARC (1976). *IARC Monographs on the Evaluation of Carcinogenic Risk of Chemicals to Man.* Vol. 10: *Some Naturally-occurring Substances.* (Lyon)

28 Tomatis, L. and Turusov, V. (1976). Studies on the carcinogenicity of DDT. *Gann Monogr. Cancer Res.,* **17,** 219

29 Wright, A. S. (1975). Early subcellular changes in various species and correlation with carcinogenic activity. *Proc. 4th International Symposium on Chemical and Toxicological Aspects of Environmental Quality.* (Munich)

30 Pesticide Workshop (1972). Epidemiological toxicology of pesticide exposure. *Arch. Environ. Health,* **25,** 399

31 Laws, E. R., Maddrey, W. C., Curley, A. and Burse, V. W. (1973). Long-term occupational exposure to DDT. *Arch. Environ. Health,* **27,** 318

32 Van Raalte, H. S. G. (1975). Human experience with Dieldrin. *Proc. 4th International Symposium on Chemical and Toxicological Aspects of Environmental Quality.* (Munich)

33 Clemmesen, J., Fuglsang-Frederiksen, V. and Plum, C. M. (1974). Are anticonvulsants oncogenic? *Lancet,* **i,** 705

34 Phillips, M. J., Langer, B., Stone, R., Fisher, N. M. and Ritchie, S. (1973). Benign liver tumors. *Cancer,* **32,** 463

35 Barnes, J. M. (1975). Assessment of hazards from low doses of toxic substances. *Br. Med. Bull.,* **31,** 196

36 Smithers, D. W. (1960). *A Clinical Prospect of the Cancer Problem.* (Edinburgh and London: E. & S. Livingstone)

37 Editorial. Insecticides and cancer (1975). *Br. Med. J.,* **1,** 170

38 Editorial. Seventeen principles about cancer, or something (1976a). *Lancet,* **i,** 571

39 Stewart, H. L. (1959). Pulmonary tumors in mice, In F. Homburger, (ed.). *Pathophysiology of Cancer,* 2nd Ed., pp. 18–37. (New York: Hoeber)

40 Murphy, E. D. (1966). Characteristic tumors. In E. L. Green, (ed.). *Biology of the Laboratory Mouse,* 2nd Ed., pp. 520–562. (New York and London: McGraw-Hill)

41 Pour, P., Stanton, M. F., Kuschner, M., Laskin, S. and Shabad, L. M. (1976). Tumours of the respiratory tract. In *Pathology of Tumours in Laboratory Animals,* voi. 1: *Tumours of the Rat,* part 2, pp. 1–40. (Lyon: IARC Scientific Publications, No. 6)

42 Dunn, T. B. (1959). Morphology of mammary tumors in mice. In F. Homburger (ed.). *Pathophysiology of Cancer*, 2nd Ed., p. 38. (New York: Hoeber)
43 Walters, M. A. (1966). The induction of lung tumours by the injection of DMBA into newborn, suckling and young adult mice. *Br. J. Cancer*, **20,** 148
44 McDivitt, R. W., Stewart, F. W. and Berg, J. W. (1968). *Tumors of the Breast.* Atlas of Tumor Pathology, Second series, Fascicle 2. (Washington: Armed Forces Institute of Pathology)
45 Young, S. and Hallowes, R. C. (1973). Tumours of the mammary gland. In *Pathology of Tumours in Laboratory Animals*, vol. 1: *Tumours of the Rat*, part 1, pp. 31–74. (Lyon: IARC Scientific Publications, No. 5)
46 Nelson, L. W., Weikel, J. H. Jr. and Reno, F. E. (1973). Mammary nodules in dogs during four years' treatment with megestrol acetate or chlormadinone acetate. *J. Natl. Cancer Inst.*, **51,** 1303
47 Stewart, H. L. and Snell, K. C. (1957). The histopathology of experimental tumors of the liver of the rat. *Acta UICC*, **13,** 770
48 Schauer, A. and Kunze, E. (1976). Tumours of the liver. In V. S. Turusov (ed.). *Pathology of Tumours in Laboratory Animals*, vol. 1: *Tumours of the Rat*, part 2, pp. 41–72. (Lyon: IARC Scientific Publications, No. 6)
49 Cameron, H. C. (1976). The pathology of liver cell cancer. In H. M. Cameron, D. A. Linsell and G. P. Warwick (eds.). *Liver Cell Cancer*, pp. 17–43. (Amsterdam, New York and Oxford: Elsevier)
50 Peters, R. L. (1976). Pathology of hepatocellular carcinoma. In K. Okuda and R. L. Peters (eds.). *Hepatocellular Carcinoma*, pp. 107 168. (New York and London: John Wiley & Sons)
51 Bannasch, P. (1968). The cytoplasm of hepatocytes during carcinogenesis: electron and light microscopical investigations of the nitrosomorpholine-intoxicated rat liver. In *Recent Results of Cancer Research*, vol. 19, p. 105 (Berlin: Springer)
52 Teebor, G. (1975). Sequential aspects of liver carcinogenesis. In F. F. Becker (ed.). *Cancer, A Comprehensive Treatise*, vol. 1, pp. 345–351. (New York and London: Plenum Press)
53 Weinbren, K. and Washington, S. L. A. (1976). Hyperplastic nodules after portacaval anastamiosis in rats. *Nature (Lond.)*, **264,** 440
54 Svodoba, D. and Reddy, J. (1975). Some effects of chemical carcinogens on cell organelles, In F. F. Becker (ed.). *Cancer, A Comprehensive Treatise*, vol. 1, pp. 289–322. (New York and London: Plenum Press)
55 Edmondson, H. A. (1976). Benign epithelial tumors and tumor-like lesions of the liver. In K. Okuda and R. L. Peters (ed.). *Hepatocellular Carcinoma*, pp. 309–330. (New York and London: John Wiley & Sons)
56 Editorial. Oral contraceptives and liver nodules (1976b). *Lancet*, **i,** 843

Commentary

Selection of doses in carcinogenicity tests

One technique is to employ the largest dose that permits survival of the majority of animals for the duration of the test – the maximum tolerated dose (MTD), i.e. an amount that will cause some toxicity, but not of such severity that an excessive number of premature deaths will prevent useful analysis of the findings in long-term survivors. An alternative is to use some multiple of the dose to be administered to man, or of that required to produce a pharmacodynamic effect, if possible the same as, or at least relevant to, that produced in man. In both cases two lower dose-levels are used also, in the hope of getting some information about the dose-response curve. The latter information might then be used to help to predict the likely risk to man, although this requires a further critical assumption about the dose–response relationship for carcinogenesis; i.e. is it linear, logistic or logarithmic?

The MTD may well swamp normal metabolic handling of the compound and so bring unusual biochemical or pathological mechanisms into play. It may also cause repeated necrosis of a tissue, with the risk of continuous repa rative proliferation culminating in hyperplasia and eventually in neoplasia. The value of the alternative approach depends on similarity of pharmacokinetic and metabolic handling of the substance by man and the test species and of the pharmacodynamic activity in them of the substance. It was argued that the use of any amount less than the MTD might result in failure to reveal the effect of the compound under any circumstances, and that careful pathological analysis of the results would demonstrate their relevance and applicability in determination of any risk to man. On the other hand, there are many circumstances in which it may be very difficult ever to administer to humans a substance that has been shown to be associated with the production of tumours in animals, regardless of how bizarre were the circumstances of the animal experiment; and yet the properties of the substance suggest definite therapeutic value.

It would be of value in understanding mechanisms if the results of a positive carcinogenicity test were not just related to the incidence and variety of the neoplasms produced, but if more functional investigations were done of the effect of treatment on, for example, the endocrine and metabolic state of the animals.

Problem of the qualitative nature of histological data

If it were possible to analyse quantitatively lesions diagnosed histologically in carcinogenicity tests, a more precise statistical assessment of the results would be possible. In particular, pathologists employ different systems of nomenclature to describe the occurrence, nature and severity of tumours. Various quantal or semi-quantitative grading schemes have been proposed, but they have been difficult to employ consistently, and they may be misinterpreted to give a spurious impression of numerical precision.

How comparable are tumours in animals and man?

Histological resemblance on its own is not always a good guide to comparability of biological behaviour of neoplasms in animals and man. There are many examples both of identical and entirely distinct tumour behaviour, as well as of types of lesions apparently restricted to one or two species. And, of the small number of chemicals shown to be carcinogens in man, some have produced an entirely different pattern of tumours in animals.

It is production of neoplastic change that is the important finding in a carcinogenicity test and not its nature; at least not until the importance of the mechanism of its production is considered in relation to other species.

Spontaneous tumours in animals

Contradictory theoretical arguments exist for doing carcinogenicity tests in animals either with a high or a low incidence of spontaneous tumours.

The issue is complicated by our partial knowledge and suspicions about the roles of endogenous factors (e.g. oncogenic viruses and genetic susceptibility) and exogenous influences (e.g. composition of the diet and its contamination by toxins produced by higher fungi and *Fusaria* etc.) in production of neoplasms in man and animals. On present evidence it appears reasonable to assume that tumours induced experimentally in animals are basically no different from those that occur spontaneously.

2

The predictive value or otherwise of conventional carcinogenicity studies

D. E. Stevenson, E. Thorpe and P. F. Hunt

In 1960 The Committee on Medical and Nutritional Aspects of Food Policy approved a report entitled 'Carcinogenic Risks in Food Additives and Pesticides' (*Monthly Bulletin of Ministry of Health and Public Health Laboratory Service*, **19**, 108). This report was short and lucid, and referred to many issues which were to achieve such prominence in the succeeding years and which have been repeatedly, and sometimes bitterly, debated in scientific journals, the courts and in the public media.

The 1960 document was revised as the 'Report of the Consultative Panel on Carcinogenesis – Environmental Carcinogenic Risks' (Ministry of Health, 1967) and the scope was widened to include not only pesticides and food additives, but also substances in industry, drugs and toilet goods. This report, although generally available, was not published, and I believe the fact that further revision has taken 10 years is, in part, an indication that it was not widely used as a guidance for test designs.

There are now several other documents which are pertinent to this topic, particularly:

Carcinogenicity Testing (UICC Tech. Report, **2**, 1969)

The Testing of Chemicals for Carcinogenicity, Mutagenicity and Teratogenicity (Ministry of Health and Welfare, Canada, 1973)

Guidelines for Carcinogen Bioassay in Small Rodents (NCI–CG–TR–1, US, DHEW)

Guidelines (various) issued by EPA and FDA for the testing of drugs, pesticides; especially OSHA: Identification, classification and regulation of toxic substances posing a potential occupational carcinogenic risk, 1977

All these documents are based on the implicit or explicit assumption that an animal study is an adequate method for determining a carcinogen. Indeed, Maltoni was quoted recently as saying 'Past improper experimentation is the only threat to the validity of animal bioassays'. I have been criticized, rather severely, for suggesting that an increased incidence of tumours in an exposed group of animals is no more an indication of a carcinogenic action than is the isolation of a micro-organism from a diseased animal proof that it was the causal agent. We need the modern equivalent of Koch's postulates, but suggestions along the lines that, for instance, mechanistic information greatly strengthens the data base have been hailed as heresy by some scientists. Plautus (*c.* 254–184 BC) said: 'Consider the little mouse, how sagacious an animal it is, which never entrusts its life to one hole only.' Perhaps we are less wise than mice, because we are prepared to make far-reaching decisions on the basis of only a single piece of information.

Until recently, the limitation on use of carcinogens was based essentially on human exposure data: β-naphthylamine and benzidine being two such examples. The 1970s have been notorious for the increasing frequency with which animal data have been used, particularly in the USA, to eliminate the production of products which have been in extensive use for many years; e.g. DDT, aldrin, dieldrin, heptachlor, chlordane, cyclamate, saccharin, etc. On each occasion there has been a vigorous and sometimes vindictive debate around the decision. Any consideration of new Guidelines has to be in the context of the essentially legalistic, rather than the scientific, interpretation which will be placed on results. I believe this to be true even in the UK, which we often imagine to be the last bastion of reason and common sense. We have not been subjected to the intense public scrutiny which our counterparts have received in North America, but we should not be complacent about this. We hope that we can retain the ability to communicate rationally on scientific issues, although it is evident that there are mounting pressures to adopt more polarized attitudes. One major objective must be to emphasize our desire to settle scientific issues by objective debate rather than by legal or political confrontation.

It may be wise to separate (a) the detection of carcinogenesis, and (b) the assessment and minimization of risk. In the latter respect, the HSE note 'Threshold Limit Values 1976' contains a proposed classification of experimental animal carcinogenesis into three classes of high, medium and low potency, and exceptions for extremely high dose-rates (which would exclude saccharin from consideration).

Carcinogenesis has recently received extensive and sometimes unique attention from scientific and regulatory bodies, due to the perception that cancer is one of the major causes of death, and that cancer could be greatly reduced by an adequate control of carcinogens in our environment. This philosophy was expressed in the 9 and then the 17 Cancer Principles enunciated by the EPA, which provide a succinct, plausible summary of the state of the art. And yet I have the very uneasy feeling that the very process of simplified logic has led to false conclusions which may prove very costly in terms both of the unnecessary expenditure of research funds and the unwarranted loss of good products from the market place. I believe, very strongly, that if our first priority is in reality the health of the general population, then we should apply our existing knowledge in relation to smoking, drinking, dietary habits, etc. There must be a cost–performance analysis in terms of research effort expended and lives lengthened even in the field of carcinogenesis. We are party to an escalation in the cost of experimentation because of the tightening of standards and the application of new knowledge. We must justify the increased investment and ensure that the reward is commensurate with the objectives of society. Any debate with anti-vivisectionists will highlight this particular issue!

The recent US Department of Labor (OSHA) document, 'Identification, classification and regulation of toxic substances posing a potential occupational carcinogenic risk' (Federal Register, 4 October 1977) expands on the 17 Cancer Principles and seeks to introduce legally enforcible rules to establish policy which need not be challenged on the review of individual substances. I cannot but feel that this will ossify a situation where the individual components are still very much a matter of debate, and I would urge that the UK does not try to suspend such a heavy millstone around its somewhat slimmer neck.

In essence the proposed rules are based on the premise that carcinogenicity is a relatively rare phenomenon exhibited by only a few of the many hundreds of thousands of chemicals, and that because man's response to carcinogens is similar to that of rodents, the finding that a substance is carcinogenic in experimental animals is an unequivocal indication that it poses a similar risk to man. As a result of the various rulings in hearings, the reliance of EPA on animal test data has been judicially approved.

You may feel that I have dwelt rather unnecessarily on the US situation. This has been deliberate, because I feel that the issues which we have to face are outlined with rather brutal clarity across the Atlantic. Among these issues are:

1. Are all animal models equally relevant to the definition of human risk?
2. Does a change in tumour incidence in an animal model establish a causal relationship to carcinogenesis in man?
3. What is the nature of the dose–response relationship for carcinogens: is there a threshold? Is competing toxicity important?
4. To what extent do individual pathologists vary in their diagnosis of

tumour types?

5. Is it possible to agree on the statistical interpretation of experimental data: type of analysis, degree of significance etc?

These provide good examples where in specific instances there has been great controversy and where the conclusions have inevitably been arbitrary. Can we learn from the past and improve on our decision-making?

I would like to challenge two basic assumptions:

1. That all chemicals be regarded as carcinogens or non-carcinogens.
2. It is feasible to reach unequivocal conclusions about human hazard in all cases on the basis of animal tests.

Thus, I am suggesting that we should be discussing quantitative, as well as qualitative, differences between compounds; and that this may affect our approach to the determination of carcinogenesis by animal testing, since the final decision may not be characterized in black and white as in the Delaney approach, but is a judgment as to the shade of risk. The approach in the UK has been historically the latter, but there can be no doubt that the former may be more attractive to some authorities. If one is to measure 'shade', then an agreed 'colour chart' is essential and any Guidelines should cover this aspect.

I would like to illustrate some of the generalizations I have been making, not by stressing the various important aspects of experimental design, but by focussing attention on equivocal results which cause so much trouble in interpretation. There are many compounds on which there is virtually universal agreement as to their carcinogenic or non-carcinogenic potential. There are also many compounds on which there is no agreement and where, surprisingly, there has been little overt study of the underlying causes of disagreement.

Phenobarbitone illustrates the case where a compound may be carcinogenic to one species, but apparently not to man. It is not necessary in this book to dwell unduly on the problems of interpreting results relating to mouse hepatomata, or indeed those for some other common tumour types such as lung adenomata in mice or mammary tumour in rats.

There has been considerable debate concerning BHT recently. Let us assume that it is a case of a compound which, by its enzyme-inducing action, modified the activity of a dietary contaminant such as aflatoxin, which occurs in a variety of foodstuffs, animal or human. Do our animal experiments make it possible to distinguish between a carcinogen and a co-carcinogen?

As far as I am aware no collaborative exercise has ever been carried out to test the validity and reproducibility of carcinogenicity test protocols when used by a number of laboratories to investigate a series of compounds of known properties, so that it is difficult to provide actual data on the variation experienced in practice.

The first problem that is encountered is that the control incidence will vary from study to study. For example, Figure 2.1 shows the expected occurrence of tumours in animals from a sample of fifty when the background is 30%. This distribution, the binomial, shows the possibility of a range of results when the only variation is due to sampling; it is likely to underestimate the true situation where environmental factors also have an effect.

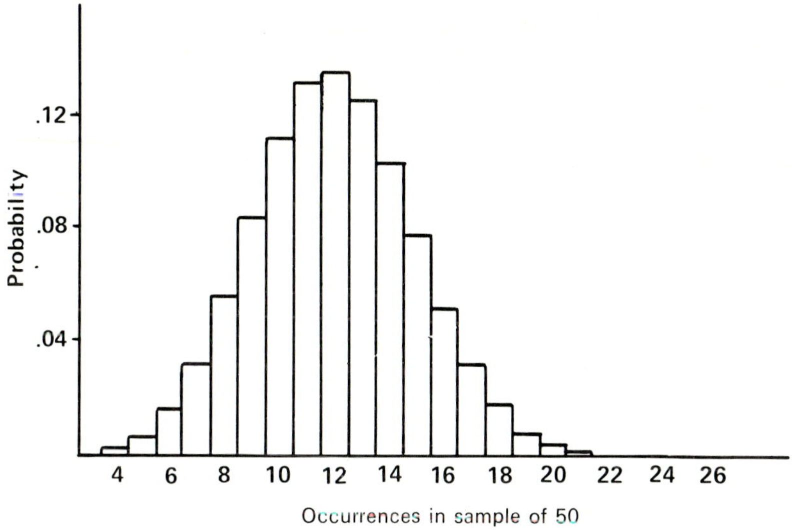

Figure 2.1 Binomial distribution, sample 50, occurrence probability 0.3

The object of carcinogenicity testing is to assess whether consumption of the compound has increased tumour incidence above background; the requirement is to identify incidences which come from distributions similar to Figure 2.1 but have a higher incidence, such as Figure 2.2 (a mean occurrence of 35%). This is the nub of the problem – the need to detect small differences in a situation which is very variable.

To illustrate the problem a number of data sets have been generated from a binomial distribution with sample size 50 and variable incidence rates. The examples simulate a typical study with a control group and three treatment levels (low, medium and high) and give the occurrence of liver, lung and other tumours among fifty animals. The total occurrence is given by adding the categories. This would not work so simply in practice, as it is likely that there would be animals with more than one tumour.

Testing 'significances' in the tables poses the next problem. If a two-sample test (control *v.* treatment) is used, then using a 5% level of significance, one would expect one test in twenty (5%) to be significant, although in truth there was no effect. Thus, due to the number of tests performed, the probability of producing a significant result is increased. If, in addition, further contrasts that are suggested by the data are tested, a significant result is likely. A further

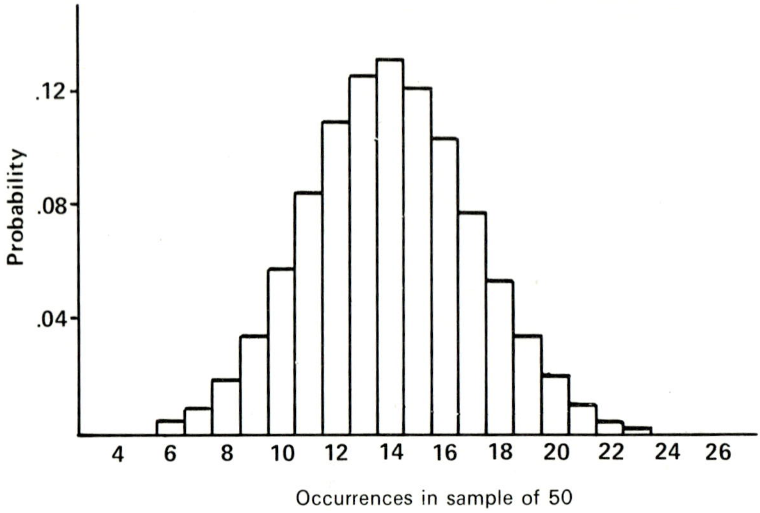

Figure 2.2 Binomial distribution, sample 50, occurrence probability 0.35

complication is that even if only two sample tests are made there are a range of tests which can be used, each starting from a slightly different basis and in consequence producing a slightly different probability.

The significances indicated in Table 2.1 have been obtained using Fisher's Exact Test.

Cases I, II and III

All samples assumed a 10% occurrence rate and hence apart from sampling differences no effects exist in Case I. However, on two occasions when the control response was low, significances have resulted. In Case II there is a suggestion that all treatments are higher than control, and if the combined treatments are tested a significance, albeit at the 10% level, results. In Case III a significance is produced.

Case IV

In this instance the assumed tumour rates were 10, 15, 20 and 25% for control through to the high dose respectively. Significances are obtained with a dose–response in the total.

Table 2.1 Simulated results (fifty animals per group)

	Liver	*Lung*	*Other*	*Total*
CASE I				
Control	4	3	6	13
Low	7	5	3	15
Medium	4	2	6	12
High	5	5	7	17
CASE II				
Control	2	2	4	8
Low	3	6	5	14*
Medium	2	5	7	14*
High	2	4	6	12*
CASE III				
Control	2	5	5	12
Low	9†	3	6	18
Medium	6	4	5	15
High	3	4	4	11
CASE IV				
Control	5	5	7	17
Low	4	4	13	21
Medium	4	11	12	27†
High	13†	12	7	32‡
CASE V				
Control	4	5	7	16
Low	4	7	6	17
Medium	7	6	4	17
High	9	4	5	18
CASE VI				
Control	6	4	3	13
Low	2	2	12†	16
Medium	8	5	11†	24†
High	16†	12†	10†	38‡

* Significant increase from control ($p \leqslant 0.10$) *for the combined treatment groups.*

† Significant increase from control ($p \leqslant 0.05$).

‡ Significant increase from control ($p \leqslant 0.01$).

Case V

All samples assumed a 10% occurrence rate, except the medium and high treatment groups for liver which were 15 and 20% respectively. While suggestive, no significance was produced. This illustrates the other side of the problem in failing to detect differences which are real.

Case VI

The control and low treatment groups had a 10% incidence throughout but all medium and high treatment samples were at 15 and 20% respectively. Appropriate significances were detected although one did occur against the low dose.

These examples illustrate the problem of discrimination between control incidence and a possibly enhanced treatment incidence if the only guide to interpretation is (fairly mindless) significance testing.

These simplified examples show that animal tests for carcinogenicity may not be as exact as commonly supposed, and that additional criteria may be required. Like other assay systems, the results should be reproducible, but the cost may be prohibitive. The combination of animal studies with *in vitro* tests also offers an approach, but this has already been rejected by some authorities; that is, in the case of an apparently positive animal study, negative *in vitro* tests may be regarded as a failure of these systems to detect activity, rather than an indication of non-carcinogenicity.

There are no simple answers to these problems, but clearly a fresh approach is needed to solve the interpretative dilemmas associated with the equivocal responses. I hope that these will be addressed when the Guidelines are redrafted.

Commentary

Biological meaning of statistical significance

Statistical tests of the significance of a difference between two groups are often misused or misinterpreted. Their power of differentiation must be considered as much in relation to the size of the experiment as to the reality of any apparent difference found. A simple increase in the numbers of animals in an experiment will not give a much more trustworthy result, at least not unless groups of several thousand are regarded as feasible.

In practice, the consequences of lack of appreciation of the true power of statistical tests have sometimes been made even worse by failure to realize that repeated statistical testing of the same or linked data will inevitably give rise to a certain (calculable) number of false positive and false negative results. A carcinogenicity test can only generate a limited number of findings about a restricted number of animals, and if the data are repeatedly subdivided and reanalysed, inevitably a 'positive' result will be obtained—on which a compound may quite falsely be labelled as a 'carcinogen'. It may appear reasonable to take regulatory or legislative action over a compound on the basis of a positive finding of a carcinogenic effect, but each test of statistical significance used to 'prove' an effect must be assessed in relation to the nature and quality of the data tested and the biological setting in which it has occurred; for example, was there an increased incidence of a novel type of tumour (very important) or a change in the occurrence of a common, spontaneous lesion (of less value without additional supporting evidence)?

Drugs versus environmental chemicals

Assessment of the findings in carcinogenicity tests, unless it be of the simplistic type that requires a total ban on any substance found to produce tumours under any circumstances, will involve some attempt to assess anticipated benefit against predicted risk.

Drugs, i.e. compounds for medicinal use, should be regarded differently from chemicals that may escape into the environment at large. The former are given therapeutically or prophylactically, i.e. to people who are already ill or who are at risk of becoming ill, and thus only to limited numbers of patients, under monitored conditions and in known doses. The latter may affect anyone, even without the recipient's knowledge that he has been exposed. This must influence the nature of the evidence required about the safety of the different classes of materials, although, as already discussed, the problems of biological experimentation are such that 'more' is often not 'better', i.e. just doing more or bigger studies will probably not give results of any greater confidence. Knowledge of the metabolism of a substance and of the mechanism of any effects it may have had will probably be of much more help in judging its probable safety.

Some practical problems of large-scale experimentation

In addition to the very considerable difficulties of housing and handling large experimental groups, the duration of carcinogenicity tests results in further problems.

It is important to ensure uniform environmental conditions for all the animals throughout the study, because of the considerable metabolic changes that are caused by, for example, variation in temperature, density of stocking, incidental disease etc.

Control of diet has proved very complex, because of the number of factors that have recently been discovered. In addition to ensuring uniform composition and quality of the major nutritive constituents, it is necessary to exclude chemicals that might influence the metabolic activity of the liver, e.g. organochlorine pesticides and other inducing agents, and to ensure that there is no contamination by fungi or their oncogenic mycotoxins, especially oestrogen-like substances and aflatoxins.

The complexity and sophistication of arrangements to standardize the health, environment and diet of large numbers of animals in very prolonged experiments are such that they are unlikely to be robust. It should not be surprising, therefore, that repetition of an experiment sometimes gives a different result. The literature and the records of laboratories and regulatory bodies contain many instances of the confusion caused by attempts to confirm or deny the result of one experiment just by its blind repetition, rather than by analysis of mechanism.

3

Mammalian short-term tests for carcinogens

J. W. Bridges and J. R. Fry

Short-term screening tests for the detection of carcinogens have recently become the focus of intense and sustained publicity. The reason for this interest is readily understandable. On the one hand it is widely accepted that 80% or more of that most feared of human diseases, cancer, is attributable to a number of as yet unidentified agents present in the environment [1], whilst on the other there is growing public concern regarding the use of live experimental animals for toxicity testing. If one accepts the view that by controlling man's chemical environment the incidence of human cancer could be dramatically lowered, and that preventive medicine should be a priority health area, then setting up a programme to assess the carcinogenic potential of the large numbers of chemicals (both alone and in combination) which are present in our environment, plus all novel chemicals produced by industry, should be embarked on with some urgency. Our present method of carcinogenic hazard appraisal, namely lifetime studies in one or more mammalian species, could not possibly cope with the number of chemicals requiring evaluation. Short-term carcinogen screening tests, because they involve a relatively brief time-scale and are largely *in vitro* based, can in principle handle very much larger numbers of chemicals and may also permit a study of the many factors which might influence their carcinogenic potential. Short-term tests are also ethically more appealing and are generally comparatively inexpensive. Furthermore, species differences in susceptibility to carcinogens are frequently experienced in lifetime studies in animals, and thus the difficulty of extrapolation of animal data to man may constitute a major problem in assessing hazard to man. The use of human material in *in vitro* short-term screening tests may be seen as a means of providing information which could assist in interspecies extrapolation.

Despite the conceptual appeal of short-term screening tests for carcinogens, it is important to consider the scientific rationale for such tests in appraising their likely practical value.

TEST PRINCIPLES

It is likely that most carcinogens exert their effects indirectly through the formation of active metabolites (Chapter 5). The formation of these active metabolites is brought about by the cell's 'drug-metabolizing' enzymes, a group of enzymes whose major role appears to be the conversion of lipid-soluble xenobiotics to water-soluble, excretable product(s). At an intermediary stage in this conversion process, chemically reactive metabolites are often produced and these may 'escape' from the 'drug-metabolizing' enzymes and react with cellular constituents, thereby modifying their biological properties. The liver is the principal, but not the only, organ housing these 'drug-metabolizing' enzymes. Much, but by no means all, of the drug-metabolizing activity is located on the endoplasmic reticulum (microsomes). Homogenates or fractions of liver, along with the appropriate cofactors to realize enzyme activity, are therefore frequently added to screening tests as a means of forming active metabolites. It must be appreciated that if homogenized liver, or fractions of it, are used they are unlikely to reflect fairly the balance present *in vivo* in cells of activation and deactivation reactions [3, 4]. In general the use of cell homogenates and fractions will tend to favour the carcinogen activation process(es) especially if the sole cofactor added is NADPH. Both the nature and rate of formation of active metabolites may be dramatically altered by pretreating animals (prior to removal of the liver) with inhibiting or inducing agents. Popular inducing agents include phenobarbitone, beta-naphthoflavone, 3-methylcholanthrene and Aroclor 1254. With the possible exception of phenobarbitone, all of these agents are likely to change the pattern, as well as increase the amount, of total metabolism compared with the situation in control animals. Generally induction tends to favour active metabolite generation rather than detoxication. Species differences are frequently observed in the metabolite profile in control animals and these may be heightened or lessened following pretreatment with inducing agents. Extrahepatic tissues often display drug-metabolizing properties different from each other and from the liver [5]. Studies with short tests such as the 'Ames test' have revealed that the presence or absence of a hepatic 'metabolizing system', and whether such a system is derived from control or pretreated animals, can have a pronounced effect on the observed response [6].

An effective short-term test, in addition to the requirement for a metabolizing system, obviously needs a biological endpoint (response system) which fairly reflects the key processes in human cancer development.

The time between the initiating event in the cancer process and the development (promotion) of a tumour is very long. Even in animals with a short lifespan this interval is many months, and in man it may be 20 or more years. Tumour induction by chemicals may be considered as three phases: a short initiation phase during which a permanent modification is made to the target cell(s); a long, multi-step, lag phase involving few obvious cell alterations; and a period of increased cell growth in which the cell(s) fails to properly respond to normal control mechanisms.

The ideal *in vitro* based screening test, in that it would be closest to stimulating known events in the *in vivo* process of tumour initiation and development, would be a characterization of a compound's cell transformation potential *in vitro* in an appropriate cell line and confirmation of the findings by injecting the transformed cells into live animals and monitoring the number and nature of any tumours produced. (These tumours should be comparable in type to those normally seen in the same species.) However, although the time-scale of this approach may be considerably shorter than the 'conventional' carcinogenicity test it is still a rather long and technically highly demanding study to embark on, and it is therefore quite unsuitable for most routine screening purposes.

The underlying premise in developing a short-term test system is that the nature of the initiating event largely dictates whether or not a tumour develops. It is apparent that in devising truly effective short-term screening systems for assessing the carcinogenic potential of chemicals, a good understanding of the mechanisms underlying the initiation of cancer is likely to be necessary. Equally, knowledge is needed of what cellular damage can be withstood without tumour formation, and of the factors which influence the carcinogenicity of chemicals. Current dogma favours the view that the initiating event in carcinogenesis is the direct interaction of a chemical, or more frequently its active metabolite(s), with the DNA of the cell's genetic apparatus in a manner which causes a permanent modification in gene expression (somatic mutation theory) [2]. Species and tissue differences in susceptibility to carcinogens are normally thought to arise through variations in the ability to form and detoxicate active metabolites and to repair DNA damage rather than in inherent species and tissue differences in DNA reactivity. Evidence to support the view that a number of carcinogens, or their metabolites, may react rapidly with DNA *in vivo* and *in vitro*, and that genetic damage rather than in inherent species and tissue differences in DNA reactivity. Evidence to support the view that a number of carcinogens, or their tumour development, although logical, has not been established satisfactorily.

It is apparent from the above discussion that an ideal short-term test requires two components, a metabolizing system and a response system, and that both should reflect accurately the effect on man of carcinogens. The great majority of the ever-increasing number of 'short-term tests for carcinogens' is based on the belief that carcinogens cause a cell mutation as the primary event in a sequence of reactions leading to tumour development, and that this type of compound–DNA interaction does not occur with non-carcinogens.

The endpoint which is determined as evidence of a carcinogenic association of a chemical or its metabolites with DNA may be:

(a) demonstration of chemical residues tightly bound to DNA;
(b) detection of damaged DNA strands or of more gross damage to the nucleus;
(c) evidence of altered gene expression, e.g. changes in cell growth; or
(d) proof of increased DNA repair.

During the initiation and development of tumours a number of changes have been observed, both in body fluids and in tissues, which are not necessarily associated directly with modification of DNA but which might nonetheless be considered as possible endpoints for short-term screening tests for carcinogenicity. These include:

(a) production and secretion of 'abnormal' proteins such as fetal proteins;
(b) changes in the endoplasmic reticulum, such as loss of ribosomes or modified enzyme activity;
(c) alterations in the properties of the plasma membrane, e.g. antigenicity, receptor site binding or chemical composition [8];
(d) loss of cellular control mechanisms [9] or changes in the cell's environment [10].

The biological preparations which can be used to simulate the human 'metabolizing and response systems' thought to be involved in chemically invoked tumour initiation are varied and include:

> Whole animals; whole animals plus added 'response' cells; intact cells (derived from tissues which contain the drug-metabolizing enzymes); metabolizing cells mixed with 'response' cells; fractions from metabolizing cells mixed with 'response' cells and fractions of metabolizing cells mixed with cell free response components.

As the complexity of the biological preparation is reduced, the simplicity of the endpoint determination and the reproducibility of the system tend to improve. However, the difficulty in extrapolating to man becomes greater, for in simplifying the preparation there is an increasing danger of inappropriately representing the human metabolism and/or response systems for carcinogens.

There may be additional pharmacokinetic reasons for poor test/human situation correlations. Thus a chemical which gives a positive result in an *in vitro* test may fail *in vivo* to reach the drug-metabolizing enzymes by virtue of its absorption, distribution or excretion characteristics, or the chemical and/or its metabolites may be unable to penetrate to the relevant response system.

Revertant bacteria have been used most frequently as response cells [11] because mutations in bacteria are simpler to investigate, are better understood and tend to be more sensitive in response than those in mammalian cells, although because of differences in membrane structure and genetic apparatus there must be some doubt about the relevance for man of conclusions derived solely from studies in bacterial systems. Bacterial screening tests are likely to play an important role in tier one screening (see p. 3–19) but are unlikely to be suitable for assessment of degree of hazard.

The extent to which it is legitimate to remove the cell's normal repair systems, which enable it to overcome many potentially dangerous chemical–tissue interactions, is controversial, for such preparations may give a very false impression of hazard if repair systems with consistently high fidelity are excluded from the biological preparation. Response systems are often used which lack the normal cellular repair apparatus, because such systems tend to be more sensitive in their reaction to the presence of carcinogens [11].

The metabolizing system most commonly used is a 9000 × *g* supernatant of homogenate prepared from adult male rats pretreated with Aroclor 1254. The use of these microsomal preparations also tends to increase the sensitivity of a test because it emphasizes the activation rather than the detoxication reactions for most known carcinogens.

Problems in assessing the predictability of short-term tests

A major difficulty in establishing the predictability of a short-term test is in selecting suitable standard compounds to validate it. The generally adopted philosophy of test design has been that chemicals can be grouped simply into carcinogens and non-carcinogens. However, an equally supportable concept is that few compounds are pure black (i.e. carcinogens under all circumstances) or pure white (invariably non-carcinogenic), rather there is a continuous scale of carcinogenic potency between these extreme situations (which may be modified by many environmental and genetic factors) so that under some circumstances a chemical may be carcinogenic and under others no tumours will arise. To some extent *in vivo* data support this view. For example, 2-methyl 4-dimethylaminoazobenzene is not usually regarded as carcinogenic, but it can be so in newborn animals [12], or partially hepatectomized rats [13] and it is positive in the *Salmonella*/microsomal mutagenesis assay [11]. 4-Aminoazobenzene has been demonstrated to be non-carcinogenic in several feeding experiments [14] but does produce tumours when very high levels are fed [15, 16]. 2-Naphthylamine readily induces bladder tumours in dogs and monkeys, and liver tumours in mice, but is non-tumorigenic in rats and rabbits; while 2-acetamidofluorene induces liver tumour in rats but not in guinea pigs [17].

The relevance of these opposing philosophies to short-term test predictability is as follows: if the all-or-none model is accepted then one can justify putting considerable effort into improving test sensitivity, as this will only lead to picking out the carcinogens. Correlations with *in vivo* data will not necessarily be perfect because lifetime test systems, as currently practised, tend to be insensitive and probably miss many 'weak carcinogens'. However, if the continuous-scale model is accepted, unless the results can be directly extrapolated quantitatively to the *in vivo* situation, interpretation of the significance of positive results in short-term test systems which give negative response in lifetime *in vivo* studies constitutes a major problem. Conversely it is a fairly simple matter to identify that a test failure has occurred if the test does not give a positive result with a compound which in several independent properly conducted *in vivo* studies has proved to be tumorigenic. This type of data is most valuable, for it is by investigating in detail the mechanistic basis for such failures that test design will progress. Such studies are necessarily very time-consuming and are seldom carried out; instead, potentially interesting test methods tend to fall by the wayside if they fail to respond to a few often unrepresentative 'reference' compounds.

In many papers on test validation, compound selection has been confined to a narrow group of related chemicals or to very potent carcinogens as reference compounds and totally bland (often very polar) materials as non-carcinogens. The approach of using pairs of closely related compounds, one of which appears from *in vivo* data to be a carcinogen and the other a non-carcinogen, is much more reasonable, although the presumption that the *in vivo* data represent an absolute reference point is difficult to substantiate. In a number of test systems insufficient consideration has been given to the need for a suitable metabolism system. This is frequently the case with tests which use mammalian cell lines. It is essential that the chemical standards used in quality controlling test procedures are those which critically evaluate both the metabolizing *and* the response systems. Aromatic hydrocarbons are atypical in that they are activated by many tissues and cell lines. The ability to form active metabolites of some aromatic amines and nitrosamines would provide a more critical parameter of the competence of the metabolizing system. Furthermore the quality of the response system is likely to be better guaranteed if 'weak' rather than 'strong' carcinogens are used as standards.

Many test systems appear disarmingly simple, causing laboratories to adopt them routinely before they have developed the appropriate technical skills and quality control procedures (see p. 3–19). This has led to a considerable confusion on the merits or otherwise of individual test systems. The length of time taken between the start and finish of individual tests is not a sensible basis on which to compare them; instead the time involved in skilful handling procedures should be appraised.

TYPES OF TEST

In most short-term tests involving intact cells a major problem is to distinguish between cell-damaging chemicals, which may cause the cell to die but not to transform, and carcinogens whose modifying effects on cell behaviour are more subtle.

Chromosomal binding and damage

If one accepts that most carcinogens are clastogens then determination of the extent and type of covalent binding of a chemical to DNA, or estimation of chromosomal damage engendered by the exposure of cells *in vivo* or *in vitro* to the chemical, may constitute an appropriate assessment of its carcinogenic potential. The measurement of the binding of carcinogen residues to DNA is an important research tool in studying the initiating events in carcinogenesis [7]. It has yet to be used as a screening test for carcinogens, although with the development of suitable high-pressure liquid chromatography systems for separating DNA fragments, this type of test may soon be a feasible possibility. Detection of chromosomal damage does not necessarily indicate a precancerous condition because the majority of the cells with such a lesion probably do not survive, and of those that remain viable the DNA changes they incur will not invariably lead to cell transformation. By incorporating into a short-term chromosome damage test a dose–response and a time–response investigation, these doubts on the validity of the endpoint can be partially allayed. Accurate blind scoring of the nature and incidence of chromosome damage is required. This type of measurement tends to be slow and time-consuming because of the need to analyse a relatively large number of cells at each dose and time-point. The introduction of sophisticated automated image analysers should remove some of these problems.

A typical example of an *in vitro* chromosomal aberration test is provided by the work of Ishidate and Adashima [18]. These authors have screened a large number of chemicals for their ability to induce chromatid gaps, chromatid breaks, chromatid or chromosomal translocation, ring formation and chromosomal fragmentation or pulverization in a Chinese hamster fibroblast cell line originally derived from lung. Findings were compared directly with those from bacterial mutagenicity tests and *in vivo* carcinogenicity data (see Table

3.1). Although they have shown an association between carcinogenicity, mutagenicity and chromosomal damage for many compounds, there are too many exceptions for this type of chromosomal aberration test to be applied routinely in its present form. Interestingly, this test system does give a positive response with urethane, saccharin and diethylstilboestrol which give negative results in most mutagenicity tests. However, urea, sodium benzoate and potassium sorbate, compounds which might be expected to be non-carcinogens under most circumstances, also show much greater changes than controls. Furthermore this test does not respond to dimethylnitrosamine, a very potent hepatocarcinogen, dibutylnitrosamine, 4-o-tolylazo-o-toluidine or quinoline. Hamster fibroblast cell lines are almost certainly deficient in their ability to form reactive metabolites of many carcinogens. The test might be made responsive to compounds such as dimethylnitrosamine by adding metabolizing cells or a metabolizing cell fraction to the hamster cell line.

Bimboes and Greim [19] have used human lymphocytes as the response system and have incorporated liver microsomes, from phenobarbitone pre-treated mice, and NADPH to generate active metabolites. It is interesting to note that some cytotoxicity was caused by the presence of the metabolizing system even in the absence of added carcinogen. The use of human material to eliminate species difference contributions is a significant development in *in vitro* testing, although for many carcinogens tissue differences rather than species differences in response may be the more important obfuscating factor in response system selection. Also, humans may differ in the response capacity of their lymphocytes thus causing difficulties in test reproducibility unless each preparation is carefully standardized. Addition of dimethylnitrosamine to this human lymphocyte/mouse microsome system, and subsequent culture of the lymphocytes for 24 h, produced a marked increase in chromosome gaps and a less frequent incidence of cross-overs and breaks. In the absence of the metabolizing system some increased damage was seen compared with controls, but in the presence of the drug-metabolizing microsomes a very pronounced enhancement of aberrations was noted. These results support the view that the failure of the hamster fibroblast line to respond to dimethylnitrosamine is attributable to an inadequate metabolizing system.

An alternative design for achieving a valid metabolizing system is to culture cells from animals which have been pretreated with the test compound. This approach has been adopted by Lilly, Bahner and Magee [21] to examine the effects of dimethylnitrosamine on the chromosomes of rat lymphocytes. These workers injected dimethylnitrosamine intraperitoneally into rats 6 h before collecting blood, separating off and culturing the lymphocytes and examining the cells in metaphase. An increase in achromic gaps and other aberrations was observed, indicating that the active metabolites of dimethylnitrosamine must be sufficiently stable to pass from the major drug-

Table 3.1 Summary of data from an *in vitro* screening test for chemical carcinogens based on estimating chromosomal damage in a hamster fibroblast line [18]

Endpoints compared		*No. of compounds showing positive correlation between 1 and 2*	*No. of compounds showing no correlation between 1 and 2*	
1	*2*		*1 positive not 2*	*2 positive not 1*
Carcinogenicity	Chromosomal damage	24	9	30*
Carcinogenicity	Mutagenicity	30	6	16*
Mutagenicty	Chromosomal damage	37	7	15

* May be an overestimate, as not all compounds were adequately examined in lifetime studies.

metabolizing organs into the blood supply. This very short-term *in vivo* test scheme has the advantage that the response system receives true *in vivo* metabolites, although it might fail to react with the very short-lived metabolites produced by the drug-metabolizing organs. Determination of the nature of the DNA fragments produced using standard biochemical techniques might be used to improve the specificity of chromosomal damage assessment in some of the above tests.

It has been argued that the estimation of sister chromatid exchange might improve the sensitivity of the estimation of chromosomal damage [22,23]. Abe and Sasaki [24] have examined 33 chemicals for their ability to invoke both sister chromatid exchange and chromosome breaks in a pseudo-diploid Chinese hamster cell line. These authors only assigned a chemical causing cals which are well established as carcinogenic *in vivo* induced chromosomal ogen if a clear dose–response relationship could be established. Five chemicals which are well established as carcinogenic *in vivo*, induced chromosomal aberrations and sister chromatid exchange. Three compounds, potassium sorbate, sodium benzoate and sodium saccharin, produced aberrations but not sister chromatid exchanges, while aniline hydrochloride caused sister chromatid exchanges but not chromosomal aberrations (Table 3.2). Abe and Sasaki's findings imply that there is no clear relationship between these two means of identifying chromosomal damage, and the measurement of sister chromatid exchanges is therefore not a direct replacement for estimating chromosomal aberrations. A number of carcinogens failed to produce a positive response in their pseudo-diploid Chinese hamster cell line, including diethylstilboestrol, urethane, quinoline and 4-o-tolylazo-o-toluidine. Unfortunately dimethylnitrosamine was not tested. Deficiencies in the metabolizing system are likely to be responsible for some of these failures (cf. p 3–7).

Several *in vivo* tests have been devised in an attempt more accurately to reflect the true contribution of the drug-metabolizing enzymes to chemically induced chromosomal damage. Allen and Latt [25] have suggested the measurement of sister chromatid exchanges in the spermatogonia of mice pretreated with the test chemical as the basis for a short-term test, while Vogel and Bauknecht [26] have examined bone marrow following a basically similar *in vivo* protocol. Unfortunately only one compound in the former study and two in the latter were employed; and none of these chemicals is appropriate to a proper evaluation of the improvement or otherwise of the metabolizing/response system interface. Whether this type of *in vivo* test will prove suitable for the detection of those carcinogens which exert their effects through very short-lived metabolites is questionable because of the spatial separation of the principal drug-metabolizing organs and testes or bone marrow. It would be interesting to see whether the latter test was particularly effective in identifying leukaemic agents.

Table 3.2 Sister chromatid exchanges (SCE) and chromosomal aberrations in cultured Chinese hamster cells [24]

	Response detected		
	SCE	*SCE showing dose–response relationship*	*Chromosome aberrations*
Non-carcinogens studied (17)	11	0	2
Carcinogens (10)	5	2	5
Not classified (6)	2	0	0

Cell growth

For many years it has been known that tumour growth can be inhibited by subcutaneous injection of some carcinogens [27]. Grasso and Golberg [28] have shown that the growth of reparative granulation tissue is inhibited when carcinogens are injected subcutaneously into rats. A similar inhibition of growth of primary baby rat kidney cells and HeLa cells was observed [29, 30] when these cells were exposed to carcinogens for 30 min prior to culturing for 3–4 days. Non-carcinogens showed only a brief, if any, inhibition of growth. Grasso and Grant [29] have suggested that the shape of the growth-inhibition plot can be used to characterize carcinogens. The drug-metabolizing capability of the cells used in this type of study is probably more effective than that of Chinese hamster fibroblasts, but still inadequate compared with normal adult liver or kidney. In an attempt to improve the metabolizing component of this type of system, Wiebkin *et al.* [31] have developed a mixed culture system comprising freshly isolated adult rat hepatocytes and fibroblasts. The

Table 3.3 Fibroblast growth suppression *in vitro* [31]

	ID_{50} in the absence of hepatocytes (μg/ml)	*ID_{50} in the presence of hepatocytes* (μg/ml)
Cyclophosphamide	> 500	20
Dimethylnitrosamine	>1000	150
3′ Methyldimethylaminoazobenzene	> 125	0.1
2-Methyldimethylaminoazobenzene*	> 250	2.0
2-Acetamidofluorene	> 250	140
4-Acetamidofluorene*	> 200	75
6-Aminochrysene	> 200	11
2-Aminochrysene*	> 30	16
4-Nitroquinoline-N-oxide	0.63	3.5

* Reported to be non-carcinogens

rationale is that the hepatocytes produce the reactive metabolites which then interact with the fibroblasts. The growth of the fibroblasts was measured after 8 days in culture. It is apparent from Table 3.3 that the presence of hepatocytes causes a large increase in fibroblast growth inhibition. It is also clear that even carcinogens which are purported to exert their effects via rather short-lived metabolites were more effective in the presence than in the absence of hepatocytes. However, this test as presently constituted fails to distinguish between carcinogens and reported non-carcinogens. From Grasso and Grant's [30] work, a study of the shape of the growth inhibition curve and measurement of the nuclear/cytoplasmic volume might improve the carcinogen discriminating power of this mixed cell test.

Mammalian cell mutation

Cultured Chinese hamster cells incorporating either azaguanine or oubain resistance have been used to detect forward mutations induced by carcinogens [32, 33]. Expression of resistance is dependent on a number of variables including cell density [32–34] presence of multiple mutant types [34] and the presence of a liver microsomal metabolizing system [36–38].

An example of the use of measuring chemically induced mutations in mammalian cells is the work of Abbondandolo *et al.* [35]. This group have used a 8-azaguanine-resistant Chinese hamster cell line employing ethylmethane sulphonate as their chemical standard. The response system is well characterized but the drug-metabolizing system is almost certainly an inadequate reflection of the *in vivo* situation. Supplementation of this type of preparation with liver cell fractions has been employed by several groups [37, 38] to overcome this problem. With this added drug-metabolizing component a variety of carcinogens, which are thought to act via active metabolites, induce mutations, including 3-methylcholanthrene, benzpyrene and dimethylnitrosamine. With some further sophistication in the added drug-metabolizing system a valuable *in vitro* screening test may well develop. Dean and Senner [39, 40] have adapted this model to develop a very promising *in vivo* test. The principle of their method is as follows: male hamsters are injected intraperitoneally with the chemical under test; 5 h after dosing the animal is sacrificed and various tissues removed aseptically, minced, the cells separated and incubated in dishes, either azaguanine or oubain added and the cells cultured for several days before determining their azaguanine or oubain resistance. The test has so far been evaluated for only three compounds. Apart from the improvement in the drug-metabolizing system, this test also holds out the prospect of picking up tissue selective carcinogens.

Cell transformation

Although the determination of cell mutations is generally thought to be a relevant endpoint for detecting many carcinogens, not all mutagens are carcinogens. Carcinogen-invoked cell transformation *in vitro* is more clearly identifiable as related to tumour development *in vivo*. A number of cell transformation test systems have been developed. Such studies are generally technically highly demanding and are longer-term than those described above. A very encouraging correlation between a chemical's ability to invoke cell transformation *in vitro* and its carcinogenicity has been demonstrated by Purchase *et al.* [41]. It is essential that in identifying the occurrence of cell transformation more than one criterion is used. Furthermore, although a number of the *in vitro* cell transformation assays show a high success rate in detecting direct acting carcinogens, they often fail to identify procarcinogens [42]. This is probably due to the deficient drug-metabolizing capability of cultured cell lines (see Table 3.4). Cultured fibroblasts are often able to activate aromatic hydrocarbons but fail to activate many other compounds (e.g. cyclophosphamide – see Table 3.3), while cells derived from embryos must be expected to possess only very limited drug-metabolizing activity because intact fetuses and newborn animals show a very low drug-metabolizing capacity.

Table 3.4 Chemical transformation of cultured hamster embryo cells *in vitro* (modified from Ref. 42)

Compound	*Percentage transformation*
A. Direct-acting carcinogens (?)	
N-Acetoxy 2-acetamidofluorene	15.4
N-Methyl-N-nitrosoguanidine	6.9
Methylazoxymethanol	8.4
Aflatoxin B_1	7.1
B. Indirect acting carcinogens	
2-Acetamidofluorene	0.5
Diethylnitrosamine	0.0
Urethane	0.0
11-methylcyclopenta(a)phenanthrene	5.8

A promising cell transformation assay is that of Casto, Janosko and DiPaulo [43]. The basis of this assay is that cultures of primary Syrian hamster cells are prepared from embryos at the 13th–14th days of gestation. Following subculture, the test chemical is added and culturing is continued for several days. Transformation may be identified at this stage from the presence of foci on the culture plate. Additionally, individual cell foci are transferred to further culture vessels and subcultured at suitable intervals. Cells are examined for the nature of their transformation by suspending them in culture medium and injecting them intradermally into the right abdominal quadrant or the invaginated cheek pouch of syngeneic hosts. Alternatively newborn animals are injected subcutaneously into the scapula region. All animals are examined regularly for the development of palpable tumours. This focus assay was successful in responding to a chemically diverse range of carcinogens, both by forming transformed cell foci which lacked orientated growth, and in producing tumours when the transformed cells were injected into animals. The nature of the tumours was not adequately described by the authors, and it is therefore not clear whether these tumours were typical of those normally seen in hamsters. However, the fact that the tumours were produced at all greatly encourages confidence in the validity of measuring a chemical's ability to produce transformed cell foci on a culture plate as an indicator of its potential to cause tumour development. From the results of Casto and his co-workers [43], the cultured embryo hamster cells clearly form active metabolites of some carcinogens, e.g. benzpyrene and 3-methylcholanthrene; however their ability to produce the ultimate carcinogens of other types of chemicals remains in doubt. If the metabolizing system can be improved this approach is likely to provide the basis for a significant test in the toxicologist's armoury, especially as the estimation of hazard to the fetus from chemicals is important in its own right.

DNA repair

In many situations DNA damage mediated by chemicals does not persist because the cellular DNA repair mechanisms come into play and largely or entirely restore the genetic apparatus [44]. San and Stich [45] have suggested that assessment of the extent of DNA repair by cultured cells employing [^{3}H]thymidine to measure unscheduled incorporation into the nucleus might be used to identify carcinogens. In their method subcultured human skin fibroblasts are incubated with the test chemical for $1\frac{1}{2}$–5 h. [^{3}H]thymidine is then added and its incorporation into DNA determined from grain counts following cell autoradiography. All the direct acting carcinogens initiated unscheduled DNA repair, whereas unscheduled [^{3}H]thymidine incorporation was not detectable using 'non-carcinogens'. Many of the procarcinogens did not invoke DNA repair (see Table 3.5) probably due to the deficiencies in the drug-metabolizing capability of human fibroblasts. This interpretation is supported by the finding that when fibroblasts are cultured with a liver 9000 × *g* supernatant, many procarcinogens do stimulate unscheduled DNA repair [45, 46].

To prevent interference from scheduled DNA synthesis, cell division is normally inhibited by using an arginine-deficient culture medium or adding hydroxyurea. Williams [47] and Lowing *et al.* [48] have introduced freshly cultured adult rat hepatocytes as the vehicle for assessing the ability of car-

Table 3.5 DNA repair in cultured human fibroblasts (modified from Ref. 45)

Carcinogens		*Procarcinogens*		*Non-carcinogens*	
Positive	*Negative*	*Positive*	*Negative*	*Positive*	*Negative*
25	2	19 (15 nitro-quinoline N-oxide derivatives)	11 (8 aromatic)	0	26 (10 quinolines)

cinogens to provoke DNA repair on the grounds that the hepatocyte drug-metabolizing system is more reflective of the *in vivo* situation [3] and cell division (and therefore scheduled DNA synthesis) is minimal. Williams [47] has adopted a similar experimental protocol to that of San and Stich [45], determining the number of [^{3}H]-invoked grains by autoradiography, whereas Lowing *et al.* [48] estimated [^{3}H]thymidine incorporation into DNA by liquid scintillation counting. In both procedures procarcinogens show increased unscheduled DNA repair compared to controls (see Tables 3.6 and 3.7). Some claimed non carcinogens also provoke a small increase in DNA repair. The DNA repair test probably still requires some further refining. For example, the quantitative significance of the results is probably reflective not of the potency of the carcinogen, but rather of the nature of the DNA damage and the type of repair mechanism which responds to it. Some assessment of repair infidelity, rather than amount of repair, could well prove to be a more appropriate endpoint.

Table 3.6 Effect of chemicals on unscheduled DNA repair in primary rat hepatocyte culture (modified from Ref. 47)

Compound	*Increase in DNA repair above controls*
2-Acetamidofluorene	+++
4-Acetamidofluorene	sl +
Aflatoxin B_1	+++
Aflatoxin G_1	+++
Aflatoxin G_2	0
Anthracene	0
Benz(a)anthracene	0
7,12-dimethylbenz(a)anthracene	++
Dimethylnitrosamine	++
Dimethylformamide	+
3′-methyldimethylaminoazobenzene	++

Table 3.7 Effects of various compounds on primary rat hepatocyte cultures [48]

	Percentage change compared with controls			
	Mitotic index	*DNA repair*	*γ-Glutamyl transpeptidase*	*Alpha-fetoprotein* (Units)*
3-Methylcholanthrene	270	253	213	6.9
2-Acetamidofluorene	120	273	159	3.0
6-Aminochrysene	213	169	184	0.3
2-Aminochrysene	120	105	148	0
3′-Methyldimethylaminoazobenzene	267	300	216	—
2-Methyldimethylaminoazobenzene	113	75	192	—

* Control value of zero

The foregoing tests can all be very easily rationalized in terms of the somatic mutation theory; indeed they may all be assessing the identical initial event. At a rather earlier stage in development are a series of tests which may be assessing different primary events or interactions which are analogous to carcinogen–DNA binding.

Production and secretion of abnormal proteins

A number of fetal proteins are secreted into serum in high concentrations in man and animals bearing certain types of tumours, e.g. hepatocarcinomas [49, 50]. Increasing serum levels of proteins such as alpha-fetoprotein have been monitored to indicate tumour regeneration following surgery [51]. Alpha-fetoprotein also develops in the serum of animals several months after their treatment with some chemical carcinogens [52–54], and its measurement might be used to detect tumour development earlier than conventional methods during classical *in vivo* carcinogenicity tests. Lowing *et al.* [48] have demonstrated that alpha-fetoprotein is also rapidly secreted by primary cultures of adult rat hepatocytes following the addition of some carcinogens but not some non-carcinogens. Insufficient compounds have been studied for this type of system to be considered suitable for screening purposes, but it does have a great potential, particularly as other endpoint assays such as mitotic index and DNA repair, can be measured at the same time (see Table 3.7).

Changes in the endoplasmic reticulum

Electron microscopy has revealed that following *in vivo* administration of some carcinogens an increase is seen in the number of free ribosomes in liver cytosol. Its relevance to tumour initiation is uncertain. Williams and Rabin [55] have developed an *in vitro* screening test based on this observation. The use of liver microsomes and NADPH in their 'degranulation test' permits the incorporation of both an active metabolizing and response system in a single subcellular preparation. Technical problems in producing a suitable microsomal preparation and in assessing degranulation appropriately have so far limited the use of this test. A similar problem has befallen the biphenyl test [56], another *in vitro* system in which a modification in liver microsomal characteristics, i.e. biphenyl 2-hydroxylase activity, is measured. When many carcinogens are administered *in vivo* biphenyl 2-hydroxylase activity is enhanced in a more reproducible manner. This enhancement may be ascribed to the induction of a liver cytochrome, cytochrome P-448 (see Table 3.8). A number of non-carcinogens appear to show a similar effect. Whether cytochrome separation techniques such as gel electrophoresis [57] will reveal a distinction between biphenyl 2-hydroxylase induction by carcinogens and non-carcinogens remains to be seen.

Chemical carcinogens have been shown to stimulate the production of pro-

Table 3.8 Induction of cytochrome P-448 in rat liver by *in vivo* pretreatment with chemicals

	Extent of induction	*Carcinogenicity*
3-Methylcholanthrene	++	+
Benzpyrene	++	+
1,2,3,4-Dibenz(a)pyrene	—	—
Alpha-naphthylamine	sl +	—
Beta-naphthylamine	++	+
TCDD	++++	+ ?
Chlorinated biphenyls	++	+ ?
Beta-naphthoflavone	++	—
Phenobarbitone	—	—

staglandins, PGE_2 PGF_2 by a canine kidney cell line [53]. It is likely that this effect is manifested through changes in the endoplasmic reticulum. Inhibition data suggest that cytochrome P-448 induction may be involved. An interesting range of direct-acting carcinogens and several procarcinogens enhanced prostaglandin production. It is noticeable that carcinogenic amines do not produce a response in this system, which is probably at least in part attributable to the drug-metabolizing deficiency of the cell line employed. It would be interesting to see whether adding a drug-metabolizing system would correct this deficiency.

Other test systems [59]

A number of other test systems have shown some promise although, as with the endoplasmic reticulum-based tests, the relationship of the endpoint measured to the mechanism(s) of initiation of cancer is obscure. Notable in this regard are two tests which involve topical application of test chemical, the tetrazolium reduction test [60] and the sebaceous gland suppression test [61]. Both tests might be expected to have some selectivity for skin as opposed to other tissue-specific carcinogens.

Summary of the present status of mammalian test systems

None of the mammalian test systems have been sophisticated to the stage where their adoption for routine screening purposes can be recommended unhesitatingly. This is not surprising because most of the mammalian tests have had only a short gestation period; to expect these tests to replace overnight long-established *in vivo* procedures, which themselves are very far from infallible, would be naive.

The cell mutation and transformation assays are the most highly advanced and now require thorough evaluation by a number of independent laboratories. DNA repair and chromosome damage systems require more development while other tests, such as the endoplasmic reticulum and the cell secretion tests, look promising but require improvement both in methodology and a thorough study of their relevance to the initiation of tumour formation.

In the majority of *in vitro* based tests the observed *in vivo* species and tissue specific response to many carcinogens is partially or totally lost. With cell fractions [55, 56] this is not surprising but with freshly obtained intact cells the explanation is not always apparent. For example, in freshly isolated hepatocytes, 3-methylcholanthrene [48] and 7, 12-dimethylbenz(a)anthracene [47], which are not normally regarded as hepatocarcinogens, increase DNA repair. An investigation of the reasons for this loss of target selectivity should prove very rewarding both in the understanding of the carcinogenicity process and in devising improved tier one and tier two short-term carcinogenicity tests (see p. 3–20). The fact that the link between the endpoints measured in some of these tests and the somatic mutation theory is obscure should not be used as a reason for retarding their development. The current concept of the mechanism of somatic mutation initiation may be over-simplified, and additional mechanisms of cancer induction are likely. In this regard it is notable that none of the present short-term tests gives a positive response for carcinogenic metals or for asbestos.

Very serious consideration must be given to quality control procedures. For example, it should be borne in mind that chemicals may fail to give a positive response in a test through being adsorbed onto the apparatus. Plastic apparatus potentially may contribute toxins of its own, e.g. styrene oxide. Evaluation of the drug-metabolizing capability of the systems used is necessary, both when produced and following storage, and is fairly simply carried out by careful selection of positive controls (see p. 3–6) or by using standard substrates such as ethoxycoumarin and amylobarbitone. The stability of many metabolizing preparations during incubation at 37 °C is poor, and the time-period over which they remain effective must also be assessed. The response system too may vary in sensitivity. For example, in cultured cells the phase of the growth cycle at which they are exposed to the reactive metabolites may influence the results obtained. Unless quality control procedures are appropriate, short-term tests will remain irreproducible between and within laboratories.

FUTURE NEEDS FOR SHORT-TERM TEST DEVELOPMENT

Bridges [62] has suggested that tiers of short-term tests are needed. We interpret the design of these tiers as follows:

The requirement for the first tier test scheme is that it should be able to handle large numbers of samples, thus relatively simple methods of rather brief dur ation which can be easily quality-controlled are desirable. In this first tier 'false positives' would be much more acceptable as a system frailty than 'false negatives' because all compounds producing a positive response would be more thoroughly evaluated in the second tier. The aim of this tier would therefore be to identify the safe compounds and eliminate them from further consideration. Tests which minimize *in vivo* species and tissue differences in carcinogen vulnerability should be favoured and largely qualitative endpoints acceptable. Because there is no assurance that all carcinogens operate via a single mechanism, a number of different tests employing biologically different endpoints are needed.

In contrast, in the second tier quantitative evaluation of carcinogenic potential is necessary, and tests aimed at pinpointing tissue and species selectivity are required. Inevitably tests in this second tier will be more technically complex than those in tier one, and rather than a simultaneous study of a compound in a battery of tests (as for tier one) a sequential scheme is preferable in which the findings in the initial tests influence the selection of further tests.

The above approach is particularly valid for screening environmental and industrial chemicals because of the large numbers of substances that require investigation. For such chemicals the development of tier one is most deserving of attention.

For biocides and drug candidates much more care must be taken in the choice of tests used, because these compounds are selectively toxic agents and are likely to generate 'false positives' in many of the simpler tests. Because the number of these selectively toxic agents requiring assessment by any one company is likely to be relatively small, and the financial consequences of making a wrong decision on which compound to develop are large, attention to the development of sophisticated tests, aimed at accurately assessing the degree of hazard to man, must be given the highest priority.

Short-term tests suitable for operation in the field, e.g. the factory environment, will also be needed for assessing safety in use of potentially hazardous chemicals.

In most short-term tests difficulties are encountered in handling insoluble materials, complex mixtures and volatile substances or gases, and the question of how to detect co-carcinogens has yet to be tackled satisfactorily. These problems, and that of *in vivo* extrapolation, require the serious attention of those concerned in short-term test development.

References

1 Higginson, J. (1968). Present trends in cancer epidemiology. *Proceedings of the Eighth Canadian Conference*, pp. 40–75. (Oxford: Pergamon Press)

2 Miller, J. A. and Miller, E. C. (1971). Chemical carcinogenesis, mechanism and approaches to its control. *J. Natl Cancer Inst.*, **47**, 5

3 Fry, J. R. and Bridges, J. W. (1977). The metabolism of xenobiotics in cell suspensions and cultures. In J. W. Bridges and L. F. Chasseaud (eds.). *Progress in Drug Metabolism* Vol. 2, pp. 71–118. (Chichester: John Wiley)
4 Selkirk, J. K. (1977). Divergence of metabolic activation systems for short term mutagenesis assays. *Nature (Lond.)*, **270**, 604
5 Bridges, J. W. and Cohen, G. C. (1978). In J. W. Bridges and L. F. Chasseaud (eds.). *Progress in Drug Metabolism*, Vol. 3 (In the press)
6 Oesch, F. (1978). Epoxide hydratase. In J. W. Bridges and L. F. Chasseaud (eds.). *Progress in Drug Metabolism*, Vol. 3. (In the press)
7 Grover, P. L. (1978). *Chemical Carcinogens and DNA*. (Cleveland, Ohio: CRC Press, Inc.)
8 Pietras, R. J. and Szego, C. M. (1976). Early membrane alterations in isolated cells treated *in vitro* with chemical carcinogens. *Cancer Lett.*, **1**, 237
9 Jones, G. R. N. (1976). Cancer: restriction of chemical energy by fatty acids as the common pathway whereby anti-tumour procedures selectively damage malignant cells *in situ*. *Med. Hypotheses*, **2**, 50
10 Farber, E., Solt, D., Cameron, R., Laishes, B., Ogawa, K. and Medline, A. (1977). Newer insights into the pathogenesis of liver cancer. *Am. J. Pathol.*, **89**, 477
11 McCann, J., Choi, E., Yamasaki, E. and Ames, B. N. (1975). Detection of carcinogens as mutagens in the *Salmonella*/microsome test: assay of 300 compounds. *Proc. Natl Acad. Sci., US*, **72**, 5135
12 Roe, F. J. C., Warwick, G. P., Carter, R. L., Peto, R., Ross, W. C. J., Mitchley, B. C. V. and Barron, N. A. (1971). Liver and lung tumours in mice exposed at birth to 4-dimethylaminoazobenzene or its 2-methyl or 3-methyl derivatives. *J. Natl. Cancer Inst.*, **47**, 593
13 Warwick, G. P. (1967). The covalent binding of metabolites of tritiated methyl-4-dimethylaminoazobenzene to rat liver nucleic acids and proteins and the carcinogenicity of the unlabelled compound in partially hepatotectomised rats. *Europ. J. Cancer*, **3**, 227
14 Miller, J. A. and Miller, E. C. (1953). The carcinogenic azo dyes. *Adv. Cancer Res.*, **1**, 339
15 Kirby, A. H. M. (1947). Studies in carcinogenesis with azo compounds. III. The action of (a) four azo compounds in Wistar rats fed restricted diets, (b) N,N-diethyl-p-aminoazobenzene in mice. *Cancer Res.*, **7**, 333
16 Kirby, A. H. M. and Peacock, P. R. (1947). The induction of liver tumors by 4-aminoazobenzene and its N,N-dimethyl derivative in rats on a restricted diet. *J. Pathol. Bacteriol*, **59**, 1
17 Clayson, D. B., Dawson, K. M. and Dean, H. G. (1971). Aromatic amine carcinogenesis: the importance of N-hydroxylation. *Xenobiotica*, **1**, 539
18 Ishidate, M. and Adashima, S. (1977). Chromosome tests with 134 compounds on Chinese hamster cells *in vitro* – a screening for chemical carcinogens. *Mutat. Res.*, **48**, 337
19 Bimboes, D. and Greim, H. (1976). Human lymphocytes as target cells in a metabolizing test system *in vitro* for detecting potential mutagens. *Mutat. Res.*, **35**, 155
20 Weinstein, D., Katz, M. L. and Kramer, S. (1977). Chromosomal effects of carcinogens and non-carcinogens on WI-38 after short term exposures with and without metabolic activation. *Mutat. Res.*, **46**, 297
21 Lilly, L. J., Bahner, B. and Magee, P. N. (1975). Chromosome aberrations induced in rat lymphocytes by N-nitroso compounds as a possible basis for carcinogen screening. *Nature (Lond.)*, **258**, 611

22 Perry, P. and Evans, H. J. (1975). Cytological detection of mutagen-carcinogen exposure by sister chromatid exchanges. *Nature (Lond.)*, **258,** 121
23 Kato, H. and Shimada, H. (1975). Sister chromatid exchanges induced by mitomycin C: a new method of detecting DNA damage at chromosomal level. *Mutat. Res.*, **28,** 459
24 Abe, S. and Sasaki, M. (1977). Chromosome aberrations and sister chromatid exchanges in Chinese hamster cells exposed to various chemicals. *J. Natl. Cancer Inst.*, **58,** 1635
25 Allen, J. W. and Latt, S. A. (1976). Analysis of sister chromatid exchange formation *in vivo* in mouse spermatogonia as a new test system for environmental mutagens. *Nature (Lond.)*, **260,** 449
26 Vogel, W. and Bauknecht, T. (1976). Differential chromatid staining by *in vivo* treatment as a mutagenicity test system. *Nature (Lond.)*, **260,** 448
27 Haddow, A., Harris, R. J. C., Kon, G. A. R. and Roe, E. M. F. (1948). The growth inhibitory and carcinogenic properties of 4-aminostilbene and derivatives. *Trans. R. Soc.*, **241,** 147
28 Grasso, P. and Goldberg, L. (1966). Subcutaneous sarcoma as an index of carcinogenic potency. *Food Cosmet. Toxicol.*, **4,** 297
29 Grasso, P. and Grant, D. (1977). Short term toxicity tests for carcinogenicity: A brief review. In B. Ballantyne (ed.). *Current Approaches in Toxicology*, pp. 218–234. (Bristol: J. Wright)
30 Hooson, J. and Grasso, P. (1977). The effect of water-soluble chemicals on the growth and mitosis of primary newborn rat kidney cells in culture. *Toxicol.* **7,** 1
31 Wiebkin, P., Fry, J. R. and Bridges, J. W. (1978). Metabolism-mediated cytotoxicity of chemical carcinogens and non-carcinogens. *Biochem. Pharmac.* (In press)
32 Duncan, M. and Brookes, P. (1973). The induction of azaguanine resistant mutants in cultured Chinese hamster cells by reactive derivatives of carcinogenic hydrocarbons. *Mutat. Res.*, **21,** 107
33 Arlett, C. F., Turnbull, D., Harcourt, S. A., Lehmann, A. R. and Colella, C. M. (1977). A comparison of the 8-azaguanine and ouabain resistance systems for the selection of induced mutant Chinese hamster cells. *Mutat. Res.*, **33,** 261
34 Thacker, J., Stephens, M. A. and Stretch, A. (1976). Factors affecting the efficiency of purine analogues as selective agents for mutants of mammalian cells induced by ionising radiation. *Mutat. Res.*, **35,** 465
35 Abbondandolo, A., Bonatti, S., Colella, C., Corti, G., Matteucci, F., Mazzaccaro, A. and Rainaldi, G. (1976). A comparative study of different experimental protocols for mutagenesis assays with the 9-azaguanine resistant system in cultured Chinese hamster cells. *Mutat. Res.*, **37,** 293
36 Kuroki, T., Drevon, C. and Montesano, R. (1977). Microsome-mediated mutagenesis in V79 Chinese hamster cells by various nitrosamines. *Cancer Res.*, **37,** 1044
37 Krahn, D. F. and Heidelberger, C. (1977). Liver homogenate-mediated mutagenesis in Chinese hamster V79 cells by polycyclic aromatic hydrocarbons and aflatoxins. *Mutat. Res.*, **46,** 27
38 Abbondandolo, A., Bonatti, S., Corti, G., Fiorlo, R., Loprieno, N. and Mazzaccaro, A. (1977). Induction of 6-thioguanine-resistant mutants in V79 Chinese hamster cells by mouse liver microsome-activated dimethylnitrosamine. *Mutat. Res.*, **46,** 365
39 Dean, B. J. and Senner, K. R. (1977). Detection of chemically induced somatic mutation in Chinese hamsters. *Mutat. Res.*, **46,** 407

40 Dean, B. J. and Senner, K. J. (1977). Detection of chemically-induced mutations in tissues of Chinese hamsters. In D. Scott, B. A. Bridges and F. A. Sobels, (eds.). *Progress in Genetic Toxicology*, pp. 201–206. (Elsevier/North Holland)
41 Purchase, I. F. H., Longstaff, E., Ashby, J., Styles, J. A., Anderson, D., Lefevre, P. A. and Westwood, P. R. (1976). *Nature (Lond.)*, **264**, 624
42 DiPaulo, J. A., Nelson, R. L. and Donovan, P. J. (1972). *In vitro* transformation of Syrian hamster embryo cells by diverse chemical carcinogens. *Nature (Lond.)*, **235**, 278
43 Casto, B. C., Janosko, N. and DiPaulo, J. A. (1977). Development of a focus assay model for transformation of hamster cells *in vitro* by chemical carcinogens. *Cancer Res.*, **37**, 3508
44 Lehmann, A. R. and Bridges, B. A. (1977). DNA repair. In P. N. Campbell and W. N. Aldridge (eds.). *Essays in Biochemistry*, Vol. 13, pp. 71–119. (New York: Academic Press)
45 San, R. H. C. and Stich, H. F. (1975). DNA repair synthesis of cultured human cells as a rapid bioassay for chemical carcinogens. *Int. J. Cancer*, **16**, 284
46 Laishes, B. A. and Stich, M. F. (1973). Repair syntheses and sedimentation analysis of DNA of human cells exposed to dimethylnitrosamine and activated dimethylnitrosamine. *Biochem. Biophys. Res. Comm.*, **152**, 827
47 Williams, G. M. (1977). Detection of chemical carcinogens by unscheduled DNA synthesis in rat liver primary cell cultures. *Cancer Res.*, **37**, 1845
48 Lowing, R. K., Fry, J. R., Jones, C. A., Wiebkin, P., King, L. J. and Bridges, J. W. (1978). The effect of carcinogens and non-carcinogens on primary rat liver cultures. II. DNA repair, cell division and alphafoetoprotein production. (Submitted for publication.)
49 Abelev, G. I. (1971). Alpha-foetoprotein in oncogenesis and its association with malignant tumours. *Adv. Cancer Res.*, **14**, 295
50 Wolman, S. R., Cohen, T. I. and Becker, F. F. (1977). Chromosome analysis of hepatocellular carcinoma 7777 and correlation with alpha-fetoprotein production. *Cancer Res.*, **37**, 2624
51 Cooper, E. H. and Neville, A. M. (1976). Biochemical monitoring of cancer. *Ann. Clin. Biochem.*, **13**, 283
52 Onoe, T., Dempo, K., Kanetio, A. and Wontabe, H. (1973). Alphafoetoprotein and Hepatoma. In H. Hirai and T. Miyaja (eds.). *Gann Monograph on Cancer Research*, No. 14, p. 233 (Tokyo: University Park Press)
53 Becker, F. and Sell, S. (1974). Early elevations of alphafoetoprotein in N-2-fluorenylacetamide hepatocarcinogenesis. *Cancer Res.*, **34**, 2489
54 Kroes, R., Williams, G. M. and Weisburger, J. H. (1973). Early appearance of serum alpha-foetoprotein as a function of dosage of various hepatocarcinogens. *Cancer Res.*, **33**, 613
55 Williams, D. J. and Rabin, B. R. (1971). Disruption by carcinogens of the hormone dependent association of membrane with polysomes. *Nature (Lond.)*, **232**, 102
56 McPherson, F. J., Bridges, J. W. and Parke, D. V. (1975). *In vitro* enhancement of hepatic microsomal biphenyl 2-hydroxylation by carcinogens. *Nature (Lond.)*, **252**, 488
57 Dickins, M., Bridges, J. W., Elcombe, C. R. and Netter, K. J. (1978). A novel haemoprotein induced by isosafrole pretreatment in the rat. *Biochem. Biophys. Res. Comm.* **89**
58 Levine, L. (1977). Chemical carcinogens stimulate canine kidney (MDCK) cells to

produce prostaglandins. *Nature (Lond.)*, **268,** 447

59 Bridges, B. A. (1976). Short-term screening tests for carcinogens. *Nature (Lond.)*, **261,** 195

60 Iversen, O. H. (1963). An early test for possible skin carcinogenesis. *Natl. Cancer Inst. Monogr.*, **10,** 633

61 Healey, P., Mawdesley-Thomas, L. E. and Barry, D. H. (1971). The effect of some polycyclic hydrocarbons and tobacco condensates on non-specific esterase activity in sebacceous glands of mouse skin. *J. Pathol.*, **105,** 147

62 Bridges, B. A. (1974). The three tier approach to mutagenicity testing and the concept of radiation equivalent dose. *Mutat. Res.*, **26,** 335

Commentary

The validation of short-term tests is based on results obtained with compounds considered *a priori* to be 'carcinogens' or 'non-carcinogens'. In fact, this argument is critically dependent on at least two enormous assumptions. First, that previous findings are at least as reliable as present-day results. And second, that the response of a given test system, like that of a population of biological test organisms, is uniform and immutable.

The first assumption is arguable because many reports, particularly the older ones (from experiments done prior to the later 1960s), were based on findings in skin painting studies that involved, perhaps, no more than about 10 animals, often without a control group. Even many classical tests of orally administered or inhaled substances have employed such small numbers of animals that they should now be considered of inadequate robustness and discriminating power, and little confidence can be attached to the results, particularly if negative.

The second assumption, too, undermines confidence in the data base against which novel methods are judged. It is most improbable that any naturally occurring biological population is of sufficient homogeneity to ensure a uniform response to any likely field exposure to a chemical. If short-term tests are employed for their predictive value, it would be illusory, therefore, to expect a higher correlation of any given test with the consequences of real-life exposure than, say, the 90% achieved at present. Logic suggests that only a battery of tests might be more successful, and then only at the cost of diminishing returns on the effort employed. The very inhomogeneity of man himself also implies that predictability can never be absolute.

As it is impossible to define a carcinogen in absolute or mechanistic terms, this property can only be determined pragmatically, and as test methods have still to be refined and developed by experience, it seems best at present to employ a number of techniques and to continue to exploit new possibilities. However, the problem of an increasing number of false positive and false negative results will also grow rapidly, and multiplication of test methods that are not based on entirely different principles should be done with caution. It is certainly much too soon to settle lists of 'approved' methods.

4

The predictive value of microbiological tests for carcinogenicity

M. H. L. Green

INTRODUCTION

In considering the predictive value of short-term carcinogenicity tests, it is important to remember that long-term animal tests are far from perfect methods of determining carcinogenic risk to man. Some of the problems of prediction from long-term carcinogenicity studies have been discussed in earlier chapters, and it is particularly interesting to me to learn from Dr Stevenson's talk how similar some of the difficulties in evaluation of short-term and long-term data are. Since short-term tests are cheaper and quicker, they need only be as good as long-term tests, to take on a major role in carcinogenicity screening. I do not, however, intend to give another sales talk on the Ames test and similar bacterial systems. I believe that such tests are here to stay, and that a far more interesting question is the influence that they may exert on the whole field of carcinogenicity prediction.

In the past, long-term carcinogenicity tests were so slow and expensive, that a result in a well-conducted study had to be considered definitive, simply because the test would never be repeated. The advent of short-term tests has meant that any result can be challenged, and new data obtained within weeks. Compounds long considered safe may be called into question at any time. The resulting uncertainty creates alarm and confusion (although when a compound is re-evaluated in a long-term study, as with saccharin [1], the alarm and confusion is probably as great.) The paradox is that whereas short-term tests were initially considered as highly artificial systems with the virtue of simplicity, I believe that their ultimate effect will be to provide a more realistic, and far more complex view of carcinogenic risk. Long-term tests may be extremely slow and extremely expensive, but in many cases they can make judgment simple (though arbitrary). We now have access to a flood of new data, and must begin to learn how to make intelligent use of it in our decisions.

BACTERIAL TESTS

Several large studies have shown a good qualitative correlation between a bacterial mutation test, the Ames test and carcinogenicity [2–4]. The exact correlation depends on the choice of compounds, which in turn depends on the types of agent for which unambiguous animal carcinogenicity data are available. A positive result in a bacterial test indicates:

1. The agent has the potential to react with DNA (almost invariably covalently).
2. If a liver S9 fraction is required, it indicates that an active molecular species can be formed by enzymes present in mammalian cells.

A bacterial test takes no account of distribution of the agent within the animal, nor of the balance of activation and detoxification pathways *in vivo*. It is specific for agents that are carcinogenic through reaction with DNA. It is unlikely to detect promoters, hormone carcinogens, physical carcinogens (such as asbestos) or agents which cause cancer through trauma. Despite these limitations, a large proportion of chemical carcinogens can be quickly and effectively detected by bacterial tests. It might be expected that the weak link in the test would be the use of a bacterial rather than a mammalian genetic endpoint. In fact the current bacterial strains are extremely good (one type of DNA may be much like another). As Dr J. W. Bridges has indicated in Chapter 3, it is probably the metabolizing system that causes most of the problems.

Evaluation of bacterial tests: incorrect

The simplest approach to evaluation of positive data in bacterial tests, is that of Meselson and Russell [5] who have directly correlated the number of mutants obtained in an Ames test with carcinogenic potency, determined by a special calculation. They are able to show a good correlation over a 10^6-fold range of potency. Although this approach may help to persuade people to believe in Ames tests, I suspect that it is in fact a long-winded way of showing that the extent of reaction of an agent with DNA in an Ames test is of the same order as the extent of reaction with DNA in a carcinogenicity study. The departures from strict correlation may well be of much greater interest, and indeed the susceptibility of the correlation to minor changes in conditions has been pointed out [6]. In view of some of the parameters not measured in the Ames test (see above), I feel that any attempt to relate mutant bacterial colonies directly to human risk represents an oversimplification too gross to be of value.

Evaluation of bacterial tests: correct

If direct correlation is not to be trusted, how should data from bacterial tests be used? For a start, I suggest that only data of a high standard should be accepted. Certain points should be insisted on:

1. Unlike long-term carcinogenicity tests, which are performed once only, bacterial tests need to be repeated. Decisions should be based on consistent results in several independent experiments. Even a statistically significant effect may be due to chance, or operator-error. There is no need to accept bacterial data until it is certain that a positive effect is due to the presence of the agent. Again, with negative data it is possible, by repetition, to place a relatively low upper limit on any mutagenic effect. It is particularly deplorable to classify non-significant positive results as negative, without further repetition.
2. With negative data, there must be proper positive controls. Obviously, it is not sufficient to show that the test could have detected a massive dose of a potent carcinogen. Not only should the test pick up a very low dose, but the reference carcinogen chosen should be wherever possible structurally related to the compound under test.

   It must be remembered that conditions optimal for detection of one agent (e.g. 2-acetamido-fluorene) may in an extreme case totally fail to detect another (e.g. dimethylnitrosamine). Such difficulties generally arise from the *in vitro* metabolizing system.
3. If a result in a bacterial mutation test is worth corroborating, a variety of promising short-term tests with a mammalian genetic endpoint are now available. These include:

   In vitro
   (a) Sister chromatid exchanges [7].
   (b) Unscheduled DNA synthesis [8].
   (c) Somatic mutation in cultured cells [9, 10].
   (d) Soft agar growth of cultured cells [4].

   In vivo
   (a) Micronucleus (or metaphase) test on bone marrow [11].
   (b) Sperm abnormality test [12].
   (c) Coat colour spot test [13].

   A variety of other systems are under development.

The most important weakness in this range of tests is the absence of a good system, either *in vivo* or *in vitro*, where the same cell performs the metabolic activation and registers the genetic endpoint. The best approaches are probably mutation in *Drosophila* [14], scoring of chromosomal aberrations in cultured liver cells (B. J. Dean, personal communication) and unscheduled DNA synthesis in freshly isolated liver cell cultures [15].

SENSITIVITY AND TEST EVALUATION

In the future, bacterial tests are likely to become even more sensitive. The bacteria are unlikely to change much, but with the S9 fraction it should prove possible to enhance specific reactions by blocking alternative pathways. An example of this type of effect is provided by harman, which increases the mutagenicity of tryptophane pyrrolysis product [16], presumably by competing for ring hydroxylation, and thus increasing the chance of N-oxidation [17].

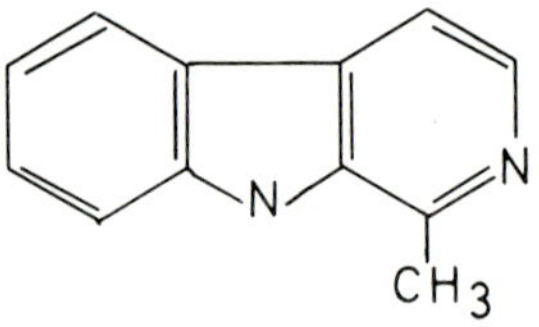

Harman

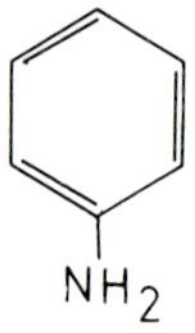

Aniline

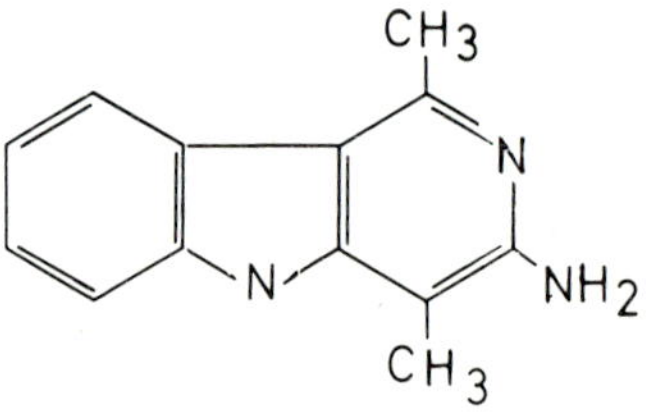

Tryptophane pyrrolysis product I

Harman enhances the mutagenicity of a number of agents, and causes aniline, which is normally negative, to become mutagenic. Other examples of this type of effect exist [17], and it is interesting to speculate how general this phenomenon may be. In a comparison of carcinogen/non-carcinogen pairs, would the greatest effect of the carcinogen be obtained in the presence of its non-carcinogen pair? If a non-carcinogenic drug contained a small amount of a potentially carcinogenic impurity, could the effect of the impurity be amplified?

A result of this quest for increased sensitivity will be that a number of compounds, which one would be most reluctant to consider as carcinogens, will show up as positive in short-term tests. This is one way in which I believe that short-term tests will influence the whole field of carcinogenicity prediction, for they will break down the arbitrary distinction between carcinogen and non-carcinogen, and force us to look at more and more compounds in terms of risk-assessment.

In my view, information that a compound can exert a genetic effect under particular extreme conditions can be nothing but of value if it is correctly used. Such information can be used wrongly, either to argue that short-term tests produce too many 'false positives', or to classify every positive result as incontrovertible evidence of carcinogenicity.

A current project in our laboratory is to assay water samples for mutagenic activity. Like other laboratories (Loper, personal communication) we can detect mutagenesis following suitable concentration procedures. It seems likely that mutagenicity is present at a biologically irrelevant level and we have to consider whether we should stretch our techniques to detect minute levels of mutagen. For myself, I would like to be able to monitor the levels of mutagen actually present, even though we may have no intention of trying to reduce them. In rather the same way, one uses a geiger counter to monitor radioactivity in the laboratory, even though it registers levels of radioactivity well below those giving any cause for concern. Indeed, it is in many ways easier to handle data suggesting a very low level of risk, than negative data from a less sensitive system.

It is not rational to aim to develop a test that will score compounds giving an unacceptable level of risk as positive, and compounds giving an acceptable level of risk as negative (no test can prove a compound to be non-carcinogenic, it can only place an upper limit on the carcinogenic risk). First, no experimental system is likely to parallel man completely; secondly, different levels of risk are acceptable for different types of compound; and thirdly, a yes/no test will give a completely random assignment of borderline cases, with no indication that a borderline situation exists.

Although a positive in a sensitive bacterial test may not necessarily be grounds for regarding a compound as a carcinogen, I most definitely am not arguing that such data should be ignored. Other short-term tests can be performed to help confirm the existence of risk. In particular, where a compound in widespread use is positive in a bacterial test, it should be possible to confirm any possibility of risk within 3 months in a series of short-term tests, rather than wait 3 years for an animal study to be carried through.

SHORT-TERM TESTS ON THEIR OWN

I have concentrated in this Chapter on the role of short-term tests in situations where extensive testing of a compound is economically justifiable. An even more important role for short-term tests is in the evaluation of compounds where extensive testing is not economic. In such cases decisions have to be based on much less information, and it must be accepted that fitting the scale of the testing to the size of the population at risk, and the economic value of a compound, will require acceptance of less accurate decisions. In product development, however, an over-simple strategy to abandon all products that are positive in a short-term test, might well lead to loss of a valuable drug.

CONCLUSIONS

A growing variety of good short-term tests for carcinogenicity are now available, which detect carcinogens acting on DNA with high efficiency. The speed of these tests means that they can be used to generate a much firmer data-base on which to make decisions. Their sensitivity is likely to help break down the arbitrary distinction between carcinogens and non-carcinogens, so that in future carcinogenicity prediction will require much more emphasis on risk-evaluation.

Acknowledgment

Some of the ideas expressed here arose out of discussions with Professor B. A. Bridges, Dr J. Ashby and Dr T. Connors.

References

1 BJC (1977). Saccharin, a chemical in search of an identity. *Science*, **196**, 1179

2 McCann, J., Choi, E., Yamasaki, E. and Ames, B. N. (1975). Detection of carcinogens as mutagens in the *Salmonella*/microsome test: Assay of 300 chemicals. *Proc. Natl Acad. Sci., USA*, **72**, 5135

3 McCann, J. and Ames, B.N. (1976). Detection of carcinogens as mutagens in the *Salmonella*/microsome test: Assay of 300 chemicals: Discussion. *Proc. Natl Acad. Sci., USA*, **73**, 950

4 Purchase, I. F. H., Longstaff, E., Ashby, J., Styles, J. A., Anderson, D., Lefevre, P. A. and Westwood, F. R. (1976). An evaluation of six short-term tests for detecting organic chemical carcinogens and recommendations for their use. *Nature (Lond.)*, **264**, 624

5 Meselson, M. and Russell, K. (1977). In H. Hiatt, J. D. Watson and J. A. Winsten (eds.). *Origins of Human Cancer*. (New York: Cold Spring Harbor Laboratory), pp 1473–1481

6 Ashby, J. and Styles, J. A. (1978). Mutagenic potency in the Ames assay and carcinogenic potency. *Nature (Lond.)*, **271**, 452

7 Wolff, S., Rodin, B. and Cleaver, J. E. (1977). Sister chromatid exchanges induced by mutagenic carcinogens in normal and xeroderma pigmentosum cells. *Nature (Lond.)*, **265**, 347

8 San, R. H. C. and Stich, H. F. (1975). DNA repair synthesis of cultured human cells as a rapid bioassay for chemical carcinogens. *Int. J. Cancer*, **16**, 284

9 Newbold, R. F., Wigley, C. F., Thompson, M. H. and Brookes, P. (1977). Cell-mediated mutagenesis in cultured Chinese hamster cells by carcinogenic polycyclic hydrocarbons: nature and extent of the associated hydrocarbon: DNA reaction. *Mutation Res.*, **43,** 101

10 Arlett, C. F. (1977). Mutagenicity in cultured mammalian cells. In D. Scott, B. A. Bridges and F. H. Sobels (eds.). *Progress in Genetic Toxicology*, pp. 141–154. (Elsevier–North Holland)

11 Schmid, W. (1975). The micronucleus test. *Mutation Res.*, **31,** 9

12 Heddle, J. A. and Bruce, W. R. (1977). On the use of multiple assays for mutagenicity, especially the micronucleus, *Salmonella*, and sperm abnormality assays. In D. Scott, B. A. Bridges, and F. H. Sobels (eds.). *Progress in Genetic Toxicology*, pp. 265–274. (Elsevier–North Holland)

13 Fahrig, R. (1977). The mammalian spot test (Fellfleckentest) with mice. *Arch. Toxicol.*, **38,** 87

14 Sobels, F. H. and Vogel, E. (1976). The capacity of *Drosophila* for detecting relevant genetic damage. *Mutation Res.*, **41,** 95

15 Williams, G. M. (1977). Detection of chemical carcinogens by unscheduled DNA synthesis in rat liver primary cell cultures. *Cancer Res.*, **37,** 1845

16 Matsumoto, T., Yoshida, D. and Mizusaki, S. (1977). Enhancing effect of harman on mutagenicity in *Salmonella*. *Mutation Res.*, **56,** 85

17 Ashby, J. and Styles, J.A. (1978). Comutagenicity, competitive enzyme substrates and *in vitro* carcinogenicity assays. *Mutation Res.* (In press)

Commentary

Short-term tests can be attacked on several grounds. To regard a particular mutation rate as 'positive' involves an arbitrary decision about the meaningfulness, i.e. the importance in a statistical sense, of a change in a population of several thousand bacteria, fungal cells, etc. Why should that particular increase be chosen as the cut-off point? And, as the number of indicator cells is fairly large in experimental terms, the chance is quite high of detecting the effect regarded as 'positive' on this *ad hoc* basis.

Many of the techniques of short-term tests involve a further equally arbitrary decision about the range of concentrations examined. It is common for compounds with pronounced physiological or pharmacological effects (i.e. therapeutic substances) to be cytotoxic in a low concentration and yet a mutagenic effect can be obtained only at a concentration very close to the toxic level. As an arbitrary decision must be made about the concentration range studied, any result can only be regarded as an *ad hoc* finding with an incalculable risk of error on each side. This difficulty, at least, can be overcome by use of the fluctuation test of Luria and Delbrück.

In some respects the problem of the effective dose range and toxicity has paralleled older experience of tests in animals. Certain substances are so toxic that it has proved impossible to administer to animals a sufficient amount to produce tumours, and yet there is good evidence in man that the material is a carcinogen, e.g. arsenic. An even more difficult problem is posed by selenium, for which there are indications that it might be a carcinogen even though it is also an essential nutrient. Imagine the difficulty faced by a regulatory authority if legal action over selenium were proposed because of a positive result in a short- or long-term carcinogenicity test.

Difficulties of equal profundity arise when a compound is so relatively nontoxic that enormous doses can be given, well beyond any reasonable pharmacological level, and a carcinogenic effect may ensue by mechanisms quite inconceivable in the real world.

These mechanisms are likely to have had opposite effects on the animal data available for validation of short-term tests.

Short-term tests are designed to be relatively simple, and easy to perform. It must never be forgotten that they may involve mechanisms and metabolic and physical conditions completely distinct from the circumstances of human or animal exposure to a substance. It is essential, therefore, to be certain about the reproducibility of any result obtained, and perhaps more weight should be attached to several positive results, even if weak, than to an isolated but solitary strong positive.

Contrary to conventional practice in biological experimentation, it has become the custom to employ repeated short-term tests in a sequential manner. As when any other battery of screens is used, this system will reveal a number of isolated and therefore unconfirmed and confusing results, but there should also be many consistent positives and negatives, to which increasing confidence may be attached, even if only at a pragmatic level.

Everyone agrees that the only way to examine the enormous number of substances to which industrial civilization exposes its members is to employ short-term tests. The health and economic consequences of an incorrect decision are so terrifying that the strategy of testing must be critically assessed in relation to the nature of each particular problem. Test methods should be selected because they are appropriate and have been validated as far as possible. Then, the number and hence the value (and complexity and cost) of those employed should be increased as the risk of exposure to the substance grows with later stages of industrial development or more widespread use. The aim in every case must be to equate knowledge of any likely risk with information about probable benefit, always bearing in mind the degree of certainty which may reasonably be applied to the test results under consideration.

The standard type of carcinogenicity test in use at present is that involving prolonged exposure of one or more species of animal. The short-term tests are secondary standards to be judged against its results which, as has been made clear at this symposium, are subject to many doubts and criticisms. It has taken several decades for the scope and pitfalls of the animal test to be realized, and it will be important that a similar amount of time is not wasted on false interpretations and misconceived notions derived from short-term techniques.

5

Biochemical mechanisms of carcinogenicity

T. Connors

The aim of this short chapter is to give a general account of the biochemical mechanisms of carcinogenesis, where these are known, and then on the basis of this knowledge to give details of some of the known variables that may influence the carcinogenic potential of particular chemicals.

A most important point is that there are many carcinogens for which there is no available information about their mechanism of action at the biochemical level. The carcinogenic properties of some metals have, for instance, been known for many years, but there is little information on their mechanism of action except for some recent work on bacterial systems [1]. Even less is known about the action of certain types of asbestos, and most obscure are the mechanisms involved in the induction of cancer by inert mineral oils and plastic films.

Much of our knowledge on mechanisms of carcinogenesis has been built up from early studies [2] on one or two organic chemicals, which has led to the general proposition that most carcinogens are really precarcinogens that are metabolized *in vivo* to ultimate carcinogens, frequently via the intermediate formation of proximate carcinogens. The ultimate carcinogens are strongly electrophilic reactants that can combine covalently with cellular molecules which have nucleophilic centres (that is negatively charged centres or centres of high electron density). Even so, there are some organic chemical carcinogens, such as chloroform, thioacetamide and ethionine, which have not yet been shown to fit into this general scheme.

The biological properties of electrophilic reactants have in fact been known since Paul Ehrlich described the acute toxicological effects of ethyleneimine, and since sulphur mustard gas was extensively studied [3,4] at the beginning of the century. Chemicals of this type, referred to as alkylating agents, have been used to treat cancer since 1931 [5], and their mechanism of action as

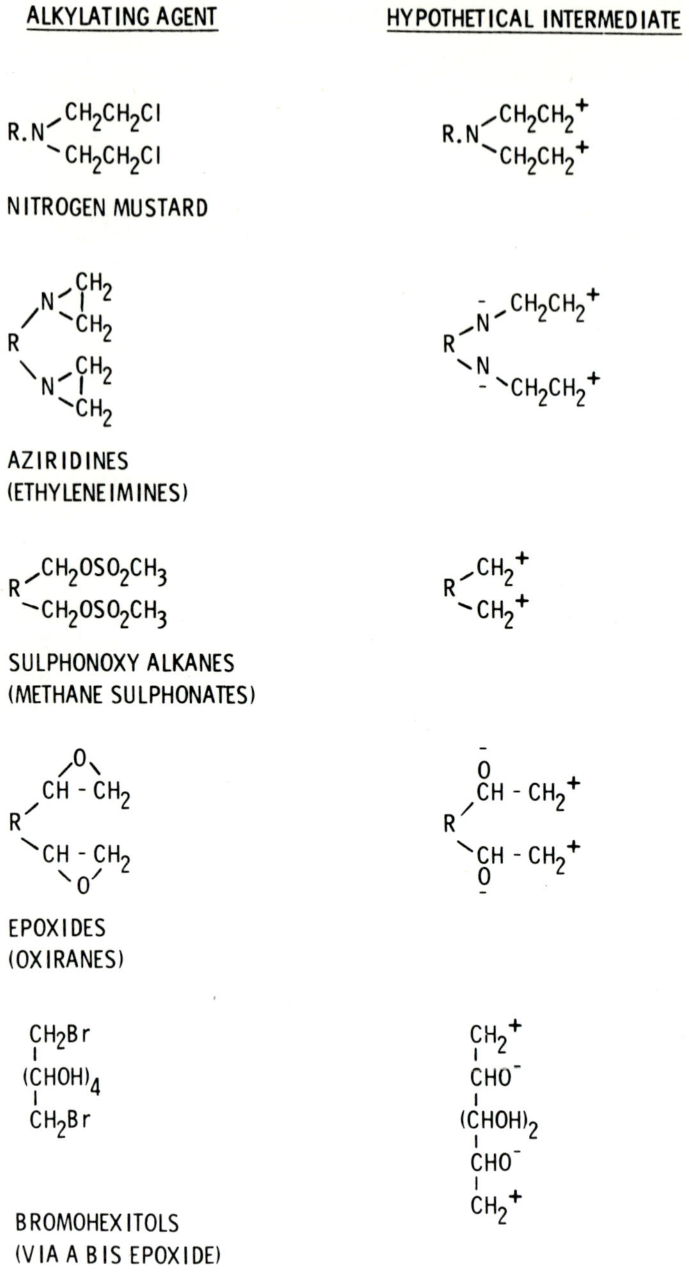

Figure 5.1 The chemical structure of some directly acting alkylating agents

anticancer agents has been investigated in detail for the past 25 years. Most anticancer alkylating agents are directly acting electrophilic reactants, although a few, like many carcinogens, are themselves relatively innocuous but are converted metabolically to electrophilic reactants (cyclophosphamide for example).

The general structure of a number of directly acting alkylating agents is shown in Figure 5.1. All behave similarly in that, on injection, they form electrophilic reactants. In some cases (e.g. aromatic nitrogen mustards), where the drug acts by an S_N1 mechanism, a positively charged carbonium ion may actually exist transiently as an independent entity. However, in the majority of cases the agent acts by an S_N2 mechanism, forming an intermediate transition complex with the molecule to which it binds covalently. The hypothetical, positively charged carbonium ion will react with numerous biological molecules; for instance, with those which contain ionized thiols or acids, or uncharged amino groups. There is some selectivity of action, but in all cases when an alkylating agent is injected, binding to molecules is widespread and will involve lipids, amino acids, nucleosides, proteins and nucleic acids. Many binding sites may exist in one molecule and in DNA for instance, the nucleophilic sites that may be attacked are ionized phosphate groups, the N–3, N–7, O^6, C–8 and N^2 positions in guanine, N–1, N–3 and N–7 of adenine, N–3 of cytosine and O^4 of thymine, while in proteins the susceptible regions are the methionyl and cysteinyl groups, the ring nitrogens of histidine and the C–3 of tyrosine. The main problem in sorting out the mechanism of action of these agents has been in deciding which of the numerous covalent reactions that are found contribute to the biological effects of the agent.

Since a lot of evidence had also been collected that DNA was the molecule most susceptible to low doses of alkylating agents, the anticancer properties of these agents was ascribed to their killing of cancer cells by a DNA cross-linking reaction [6]. This explanation is still accepted nowadays, although other mechanisms of killing cancer cells by alkylation must exist, since more recently a number of monofunctional alkylating agents, which cannot cross-link DNA, have been shown to be effective anticancer agents. Even bifunctional alkylating agents do not necessarily cross-link DNA strands. Figure 5.2 shows that besides cross-linking adjacent strands of DNA, cross links may be formed in the same strand or between DNA and protein. In addition, many monofunctional alkylations will occur, the second electrophilic arm reacting with water. The mechanism of cell death is not known, but is thought to be by a process of 'unbalanced growth' analogous to thymineless death observed in bacteria. Alkylation of cells in the mitotic cycle interferes specifically with DNA synthesis and has little or no effect on RNA or protein synthesis. This in an unknown way leads to cell death via the formation of giant cells with abnormal ratios of macromolecules, which is a common finding in cells treated with alkylating agents. It is also certain that at lower dose-levels there may be damage to DNA but not cell death. It has been known for many years that alkylating agents used in the treatment of cancer can also cause cancer, and the connection between the two is that probably at high doses these agents kill cells by excessive DNA damage, while at lower doses there is sub-lethal DNA damage, which in some way leads to the altered

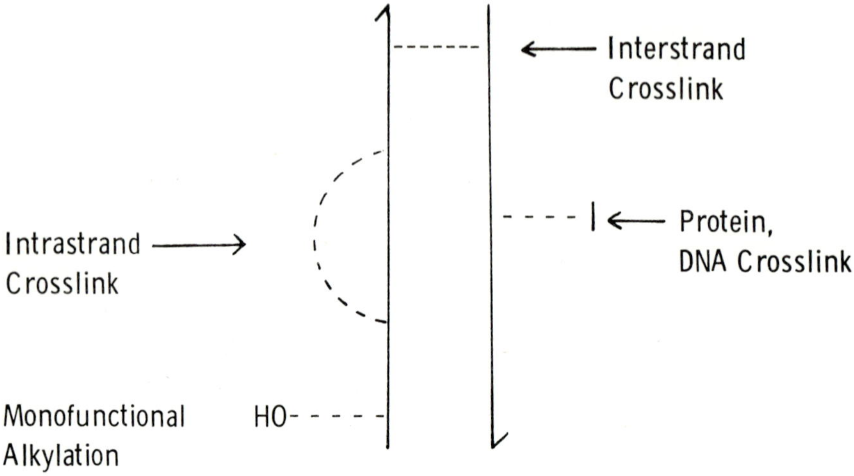

Figure 5.2 Types of reaction occurring between DNA and difunctional alkylating agents

gene expression necessary for malignancy. It has also been known for a long time that carcinogens which are not electrophilic reactants *per se* also have anticancer properties (e.g. polycyclic hydrocarbons), but it was not suggested at the time that their properties might be due to their conversion *in vivo* to reactive alkylating metabolites.

METABOLISM OF ACETYLAMINOFLUORENE

The first suggestion that carcinogens might require activation *in vitro* before they could exert their effects came from extensive studies on the animal hepatocarcinogen acetylaminofluorene (AAF). The pathways involved in the metabolism of this chemical are shown in Figure 5.3. On ingestion AAF is metabolized mainly by the microsomal mixed function oxidases of the liver. The major metabolites are ring hydroxylation products and their conjugates which are not chemically reactive (Figure 5.3; 1). However, in addition to this detoxification reaction, a small amount of the N-hydroxy derivative is formed (N-hydroxy AAF Figure 5.3; 2). A major fraction of N-hydroxy AAF is converted to the O-glucuronide (Figure 5.3; 3), which has only weak electrophilic activity, but if it were converted to its de-acetylated derivative a strong electrophile would be formed. The animals most susceptible to AAF-induced carcinogenesis have high levels of sulphotransferase enzymes in their liver, which can convert N-hydroxy AAF to its unstable O-sulphate (Figure 5.3; 4). This conjugate can break down to a very powerful electrophilic reactant. Because of this finding and similar correlations the sulphate ester is generally considered to be the major carcinogenic metabolite of AAF. There also exists in liver and extrahepatic tissues, acyltransferase enzymes which can transfer the acetyl group of N-hydroxy AAF to the oxygen atom of the corresponding hydroxylamine [7]. This derivative (Figure 5.3; 5) is also a very strong electrophile and may explain the mechanism of cancer induction by AAF in extrahepatic tissues. Another recent finding has been that peroxidases may act on AAF to form free radicals (Figure 5.3; 6) which can act in a similar way to electrophilic reactants formed by heterolytic fission. The picture is thus a very complex one, with AAF being converted under particular conditions to a variety of products some of which are chemically unreactive and likely to be excreted. Others are weak electrophilic reactants, which may undergo further metabolism to strong electrophilic reactants, and still others are powerful electrophilic reactants in their own right.

OTHER AROMATIC AMINES

Similar pathways have been shown to exist for other types of aromatic amines, such as the aminoazobenzenes, naphthylamines and aminobiphenyls. Failure to activate a compound, for example the poor N-hydroxylation of 1-naphthylamine, can explain why some aromatic amines are not carcinogenic, whereas closely related structures are. Any aromatic amine, unless proved otherwise, should be suspected as a carcinogen. Unfortunately, although the pathways of metabolism of aromatic amines are broadly similar they are not identical, and this prevents the design of a simple '*in vitro*' biochemical test for the detection of carcinogenic amines.

N, N-dimethylaminoazobenzene is, like AAF, a liver carcinogen, and after demethylation it is similarly N-hydroxylated and esterified by liver sulphotransferase. However, N-hydroxylation of methylaminoazobenzene is not, as is the case for AAF, mediated by cytochrome P450-dependent enzymes but by an NADPH-requiring flavoprotein [8]. 4-nitroquinoline-1-oxide is reduced to 4 hydroxyaminoquinoline-1-oxide and subsequently esterified to an electrophilic reactant. In this case, however, the hydroxylamine is esterified by seryl-tRNA [9]. The different types of reactive esters formed, and the different pathways by which they are formed, could certainly be responsible

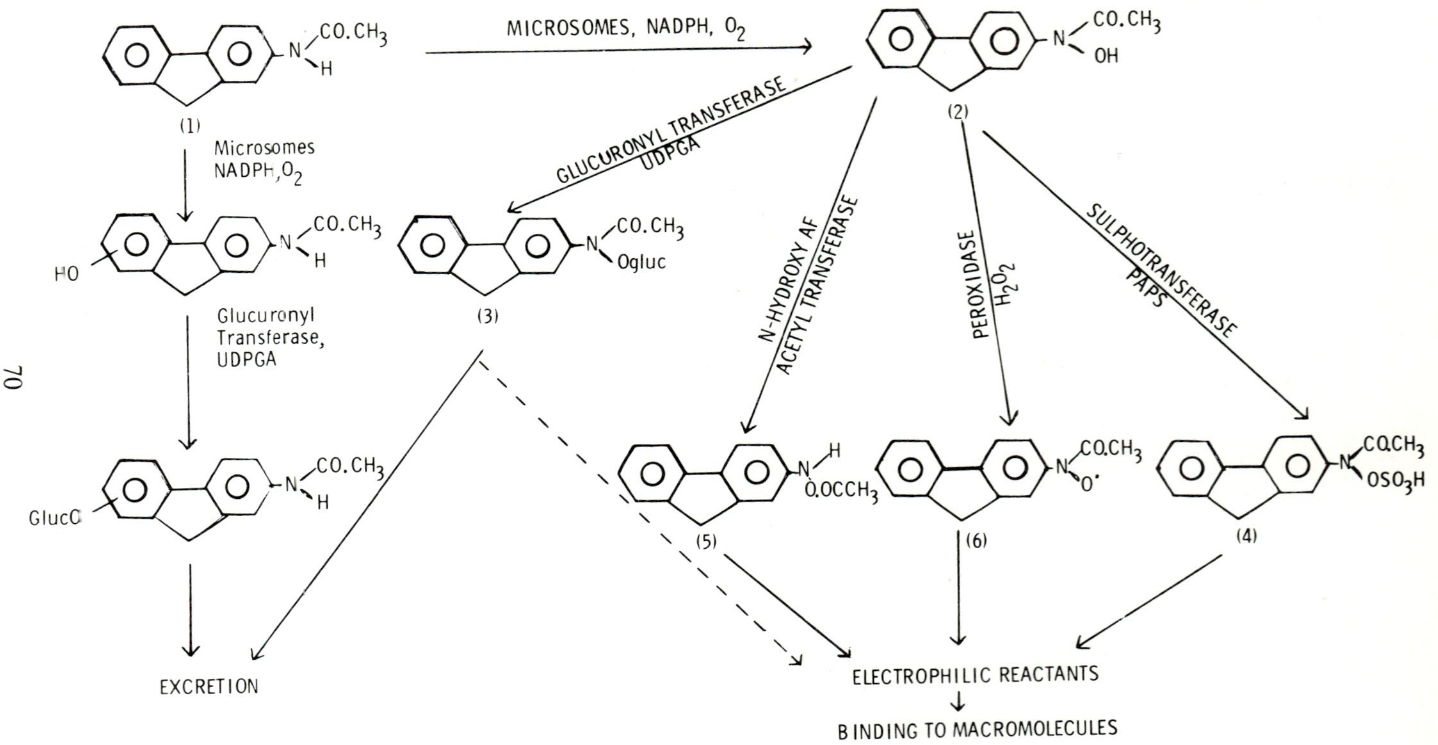

Figure 5.3 Metabolic pathways of acetylaminofluorene

for large differences in potency, species susceptibility and organ specificity. β-naphthylamine and 4-aminobiphenyl are potent carcinogens and are activated like AAF after esterification of the corresponding hydroxylamine. But AAF is a liver carcinogen and these two chemicals are bladder carcinogens. The difference may be the result of the formation of the N-glucuronides of the two bladder carcinogens. Formed in the liver, the N-glucuronides enter the circulation and accumulate in the bladder. In this acid environment protonation may take place and the resulting nitrenium ions may be the ultimate carcinogens. It is by no means clear why some hydroxylamines should be converted to their O-sulphates and be liver carcinogens (because of their instability), while others are converted to their N-glucuronides which being more stable may be transported to the bladder which is the target tissue. Because of these variations it is not possible to make accurate predictions of the likely carcinogenic potency of an amine or of its organ-specificity.

OTHER WAYS OF FORMING ELECTROPHILIC REACTANTS

A large variety of chemical structures may be metabolized by different pathways to electrophilic reactants of different types (Figure 5.4). Benz(a)pyrene has been studied in particular detail and can be converted by different pathways to numerous metabolites, usually via initial formation of an epoxide [10]. Diol epoxides and, in particular, isomeric vicinal diol epoxides derived from benzo(a)pyrene 7,8-dihydrodiols appear to be particularly important [11]. Epoxidation of double bonds is a common mechanism of activation of procarcinogens and this process is probably involved in the carcinogenicity of chemicals such as safrole (and related flavouring agents) and aflatoxin B_1 (Figure 5.4). Dealkylation leading to an unstable complex whose ultimate fate is breakdown to electrophilic reactants is also a common mechanism, and is involved in the carcinogenicity of the dialkyl triazenes, some nitrosamines and the chemotherapeutic agent natulan (Figure 5.4). Other mechanisms are represented by the activation pathways of pyrrolizidine alkaloids (Figure 5.4), ethionine and hydrazines. It has recently been shown that vinyl carbamate is a more potent carcinogen than ethyl carbamate (urethane) and it has been proposed that it may be the carcinogenic metabolite of urethane. If this is the case, it may be argued that almost any saturated aliphatic compound may be converted to a carcinogen by the introduction of a double bond into the molecule. As it has already been demonstrated that aliphatic and aromatic double bonds may be activated by epoxidation, then almost any

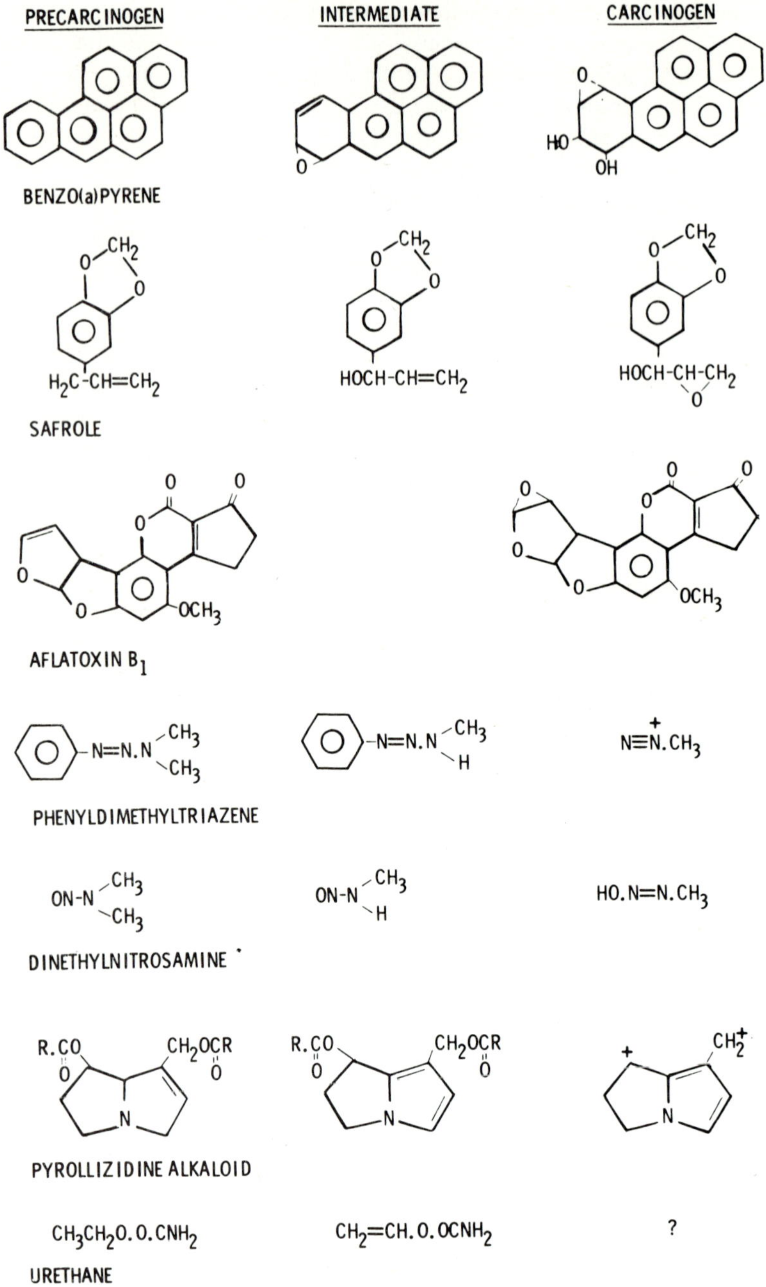

Figure 5.4 Proposed activation pathways of some animal carcinogens

organic chemical has the potential to be activated, at least in theory, to a carcinogen.

FACTORS INFLUENCING CARCINOGENESIS

Figure 5.5 shows just some of the factors that can influence the formation of an electrophilic reactant from a precarcinogen, or which can influence the development of cancer following covalent binding of the reactant with its 'target' nucleophile. The level of exposure to the carcinogen is very important, since it has been shown that the type of conjugate formed may be dependent on the serum concentration of the chemical. If at low doses glucuronides are formed exclusively and sulphates only at high dose-levels, then in the case of carcinogens activated by sulphate esterification a 'safe' concentration may exist. This also means that one cannot predict, from the effects of a high dose-level of a carcinogen, the effects that may result from a low dose-level or from chronic exposure. The complexity of metabolic pathways for individual chemicals has already been described, and hence any factor which alters the quality or quantity of drug metabolism, especially in liver microsomes, will influence the carcinogenic potential of a procarcinogen. Factors such as animal strain, species, hormonal status, age, sex, diet and the presence of microsomal inhibitors or inducers may all profoundly affect the ability of a chemical to cause cancer. Dietary constituents may be important in other ways. Nitrosamines may be formed endogenously from the interaction of nitrites and amines in the gastrointestinal tract, which may lead to conflicting results if this process were to occur to a large extent during examination of another carcinogen. The diet may also contain significant amounts of other carcinogens, co-carcinogens and promoters and so it, too, may similarly affect the outcome of experiments designed to assess the carcinogenicity of a chemical. Butylated N-hydroxyanisole, an antioxidant, can greatly reduce the binding of activated benzpyrene metabolites to DNA and increase the detoxification of N-hydroxy AAF by enhancing glucuronic acid conjugation. In both cases it is likely that there is protection against the carcinogenic action of these chemicals [12,13]. Disulfiram and related chemicals can inhibit cancer induced by dimethylhydrazine. In this case activation of the carcinogen is prevented by a reactive metabolite of disulfiram inhibiting microsomal function. A wide variety of naturally occurring constituents have been found which can similarly reduce activation of carcinogens. On the other hand, other dietary constituents may stimulate the production of electrophilic reactants by directly influencing microsomes, or by competing with the carcinogen for detoxification pathways and increasing the amount metabolized by activating pathways.

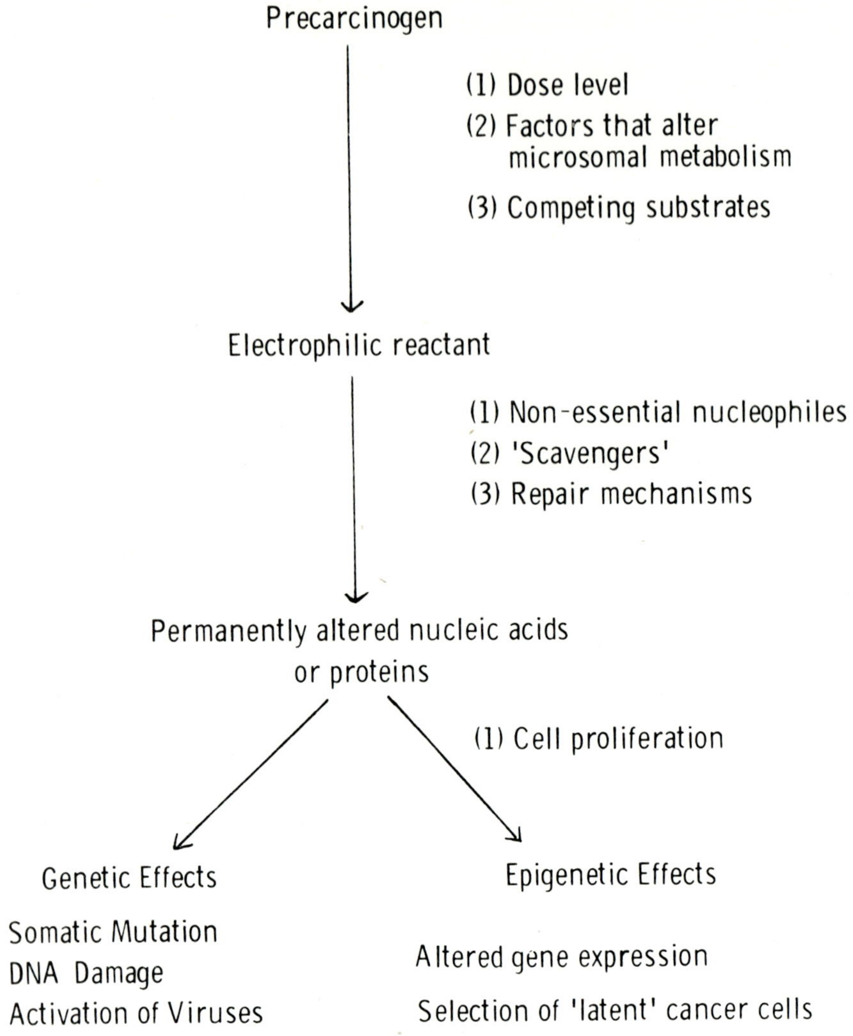

Figure 5.5 Some of the variables involved in chemical carcinogenesis

Once formed the electrophilic reactant may bind to any number of molecules, some of which may be non-essential, and others which are in such high concentration that the relatively small amount of inactivation that takes place is of no great consequence. It is in fact quite simple to protect cells from the acute cytotoxic effects of electrophilic reactants by treatment with powerful nucleophiles, such as cysteine, which have a high competition factor and greatly reduce binding to macromolecules.

Even after the electrophile has reacted sufficiently with its 'target' molecule, whether or not a cancer will ultimately develop is dependent on variables such as the stage of the cell cycle at the time of binding, DNA (and perhaps other) repair mechanisms, the stimulation of cell proliferation and probably a whole host of other unknown factors.

EXTRAPOLATION TO MAN

It is likely that many more chemicals thought to be harmless will one day be shown to be potentially carcinogenic in man because they can be converted by metabolism to reactive metabolites. However, while a compound may be labelled 'potentially carcinogenic' because of the way it is handled *in vivo*, or because of its analogy to known carcinogens, it is difficult to make a quantitative extrapolation to man because of the numerous variables described above. If a chemical is a highly reactive electrophilic reactant *per se* then it should be treated as a dangerous carcinogen, e.g. sulphur mustard which is known to be carcinogenic in animals and man. Similarly, if a chemical can be shown to be metabolized in animals to a large extent to an electrophilic reactant, then again it should be treated as a carcinogen for man. An example of this class of compound would be aflatoxin B_1, which is rapidly and exclusively metabolized to an electrophilic reactant in a variety of species. There is in fact strong presumptive evidence from epidemiological studies that aflatoxins are carcinogenic for man. The major metabolic pathways for the nitrosamines and dialkyl triazenes are activating ones, and these should also be treated as dangerous carcinogens. Unfortunately for the majority of animal carcinogens there are a series of complicated metabolic pathways and only a few minor ones may be responsible for the generation of ultimate carcinogens. It is not unreasonable to assume that dose-levels of exposure may exist where no electrophilic reactants are formed and where there is no risk of cancer induction. Unfortunately it is impossible to test this hypothesis experimentally, because it is not feasible (because of the numbers involved) to carry out experiments on animals at low dose-levels of carcinogens in order to establish the shape of the dose–response curve.

It is reasonable to assume that most dangerous organic chemical carcinogens should now be readily detectable. Such chemicals should show activity at low concentrations in short-term screening tests which measure some form of DNA damage, and might be expected to be converted to electrophilic reactants by a major metabolic pathway. However, some chemicals can only be shown to be active in short-term screening tests by using highly sensitive methods. They may also only produce minute amounts of electrophilic reactants during metabolism. It could still be argued that these chemicals must still be treated as carcinogens, since any concentration of an electrophilic reactant, however small, may cause a malignant change. A counter-argument would be that under normal conditions of exposure, the chances of an electrophilic reactant being formed, or of its ever binding to a significant extent to the target molecule, are so remote that it should not be considered to be a hazardous substance.

The decision to continue to use such a chemical cannot depend on scientific arguments alone because these are equivocal, but on some other wider form of judgment taking into consideration the 'social' value of the chemical.

References

1 Venitt, S. and Levy, L. S. (1974): Mutagenicity of chromates in bacteria and its relevance to chromate carcinogenesis. *Nature (Lond.)* **250,** 493

2 Miller, J. A. (1970). Carcinogenesis by chemicals: an overview. (G. H. A. Clowes, Memorial Lecture). *Cancer Res.*, **30,** 559

3 Lynch, V., Smith, M. W. and Marshall, E. K. (1918). Dichloroethyl sulfide. Mustard gas. I. The systemic effects and mechanism of action. *J. Pharmacol. Exp. Therap.*, **12,** 265

4 Krumbhaar, E.B. and Krumbhaar, H.D. (1919). The blood and bone marrow in mustard gas poisoning. *J. Med. Res.*, **40,** 497

5 Adair, F. E. and Bagg, H. J. (1931). Experimental and clinical studies on the treatment of cancer by dichloroethylsulfide. *Ann. Surg.*, **93,** 190

6 Lawley, P. D. and Brookes, P. (1967). Interstrand cross linking of DNA by difunctional alkylating agents. *J. Molec. Biol.*, **25,** 143

7 King, C. M. and Olive, C. W. (1975). Comparative effects of strain, species and sex on the acyltransferase and sulfotransferase catalyzed activation of N-hydroxy-N-2-fluorenylacetamide. *Cancer Res.*, **35,** 906

8 Kadlubar, F. F., Miller, J. A., Miller, E. C. (1976). Microsomal N-oxidation of the hepatocarcinogen, 4N-methyl-4-aminoazobenzene. *Cancer Res.*, **36,** 1196

9 Tada, M. and Tada, M. (1976). Metabolic activation of 4-nitroquinoline-1-oxide and its binding to nucleic acid. In P. N. Magee, S. Takayama, T. Sugimura and T. Matsushima (eds.). *Fundamentals of Cancer Prevention*, pp. 217–227. (Baltimore: University Park Press)

10 Dipple, A. (1976). Polynuclear aromatic carcinogens. In C. E. Searle, (ed.). *Chemical Carcinogenesis*. Amer. Chem. Soc. Monogr. No. 173, pp. 245–300 (Washington)

11 Yang, S. K., McCourt, D. W., Leutz, J. C. and Gelboin, H. V. (1977) Benzo(a)pyrene diol epoxides: mechanism of enzymatic formation and optically active intermediates. *Science*, **196,** 1199

12 Lam, L. K. T. and Wattenberg, L. W. (1977). Effects of butylated hydroxyanisole on the metabolism of benzo(a)pyrene by mouse liver microsomes. *J. Natl Cancer Inst.*, **58,** 413

13 Grantham, P. H., Weisburger, J. H. and Weisburger, E. K. (1973). Effects of the antioxidant butylated hydroxytoluene on the metabolism of the carcinogens N-2-fluorenylacetamide and N-hydroxy-N-2-fluorenylacetamide *Food Cosmet. Toxicol.*, **11,** 209

14 Ehrlich, P. (1956). *Collected Papers of Paul Ehrlich* (ed. F. Himmelweit), pp 596–618 (London: Pergamon Press)

Commentary

A basic uncertainty that affects all our consideration of mechanisms and tests of carcinogenicity is that hardy problem of pathology – the definition of a carcinogen. It may not be difficult to agree that a strong carcinogen is a chemical of which a small amount causes rapid development of many malignant tumours, but as was discussed elsewhere at this meeting, it is far harder to define lesser effects in a consistent and reproducible fashion.

The variety of biochemical mechanisms directly involved in the production of carcinogenic molecules, as well as in their detoxification and removal, means that there are many points at which even quite subtle influences may turn a substance from, say in simplistic terms, a non-carcinogen to a carcinogen. This shows how important it is to support the result of one test with others. It is just as necessary to consider the possible biochemical mechanism of action and how realistic it is to expect it to occur in man.

6

The economics of carcinogenicity testing

D. M. Conning

Although the death rate per million population is tending to decline in the UK, the overall death rate from cancer is increasing (Figure 6.1) and the increase is matched, curiously, by the rate of increase of fixed assets in the chemical industry over the same period of time (1969–1973). This has suggested to some that the increased ability of the industry to manufacture chemicals is correlated with a rise in the cancer rate. The correlation is not real because the major part of the rise in cancer rates is due to pulmonary tumours resulting from cigarette smoking, and other tumour rates are very variable according to geographical and biological location. There is thus no real relationship between overall death rates from cancer and the activity of the chemical industry. Nevertheless, that governments think otherwise is shown by the rate of expenditure on toxicological clearance studies that need to be undertaken by a company such as ICI Limited (Figure 6.1) to satisfy regulatory requirements. Of course, the chemical industry is a neatly definable, easily regulable entity with a fearsome reputation for pollution, and thus a ready source of political bonus points – but at what cost, in the long run, to an industrial society such as our own?

In considering the economic impact of these toxicological constraints, in particular those relating to carcinogenicity, I have made three assumptions:

1. People should be protected against the risk of occupational cancer.
2. Chemicals which cause cancer may be produced, if proper safeguards are taken.
3. A reasonably sound prediction of a cancer risk to man is possible from animal studies.

First, that people should be protected against the risk of occupational cancer in the work-place. In an advanced affluent society this means that all available safeguards in terms of plant design and protective clothing will be taken when the possibility is identified that a chemical has carcinogenic potential. Making this assumption avoids the problems of risk/benefit analyses which are probably irrelevant in the present context. If the debate is broadened to include all aspects of human and environmental toxicology, the question of benefit would assume a much more important role.

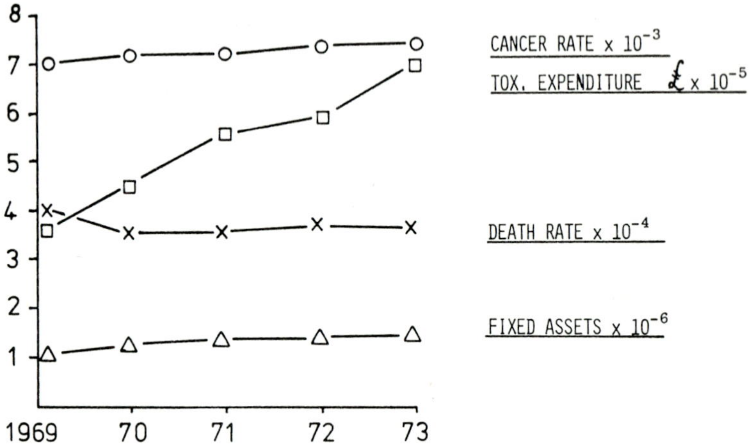

Figure 6.1 Overall death rates, and death rates from cancer, compared with investment in chemical plant and on safety evaluation in pounds of the year

The second assumption is that there will be no automatic bar to the production of a chemical because it is identified as a potential human carcinogen. It is taken as axiomatic that all proper safeguards will be taken. By making this assumption, we can avoid considering the economic consequences to society of an outright ban on production – a topic fraught with unpredictable variables.

The third assumption is that, given enough resources, it is reasonable to expect a toxicologist to be able to decide that a chemical will cause cancer in man when the circumstance of dosage and route of exposure are correct. This begs the questions of experimental design and the difficulties of statistical analysis, the influence of diet and nutrition, the route of administration, and assumes these problems can be overcome by adequate allocation of time and money.

ECONOMICS OF CARCINOGENICITY TESTING

The total cost of controlling the use of a carcinogen includes, in addition to the cost of testing, the cost of designing and installing manufacturing equipment to ensure safe production, and the cost of monitoring the work force to ensure production is indeed safe (Table 6.1). The cost of carcinogenicity testing varies according to the intensity of the work involved, which will itself depend on the physical properties of the material, the industrial process to be employed and the numbers of people who would be at risk. Similarly, the capital cost of rendering the manufacturing plant safe to operate will vary according to these same factors, and to the scale of operation. It is assumed the additional capital costs would rarely exceed 10% of the total.

Table 6.1 Cost of cancer testing and monitoring

1. TEST COSTS	
Two or three animal species	
Two routes of administration	
Three dose-levels	£0·2 m–0·6 m
Purified diets	
Expert analyses, etc.	
In utero + three generation cytogenetics	£0·25 m
Total £0·2 m–0·85 m	
Average £0·5 m	
2. CAPITAL COSTS	
Marginal cost of safe production – 1–10%	
3. HUMAN MONITORING COSTS	
Routine screening of each worker	
Approx. £1000 per annum.	
Average per modern plant £0·2 m per annum.	

Human monitoring refers specifically to screening of the work force for the development of the relevant tumours as defined by the animal studies. This assumes it will be possible in future to devise procedures which allow the recognition that hazardous exposure has occurred, thus enabling redeployment of the worker before irreversible disease ensues. It is recognized that such screening is perhaps largely a theoretical possibility at present, but costs roughly of £1000 per person per annum seem a reasonable estimate, based on the assumption that the procedures will not differ radically from current health screening procedures.

These figures do not include the capital investment which would be necessary to provide the requisite animal testing facilities and laboratories to undertake the human screening procedures. Such an investment would be in the region of £100 million but, because it would be expenditure over a limited period of time and not a continuing burden on manufacturing industry, it is excluded from the present arguments.

In order to place the testing and monitoring costs in some sort of perspective, it is necessary to examine the total costs of research, development and production which currently pertain, and to examine the place that the test and control programme holds (Figure 6.2). Products vary in the length of time which elapses between the discovery and the 'break-even' point; and in the

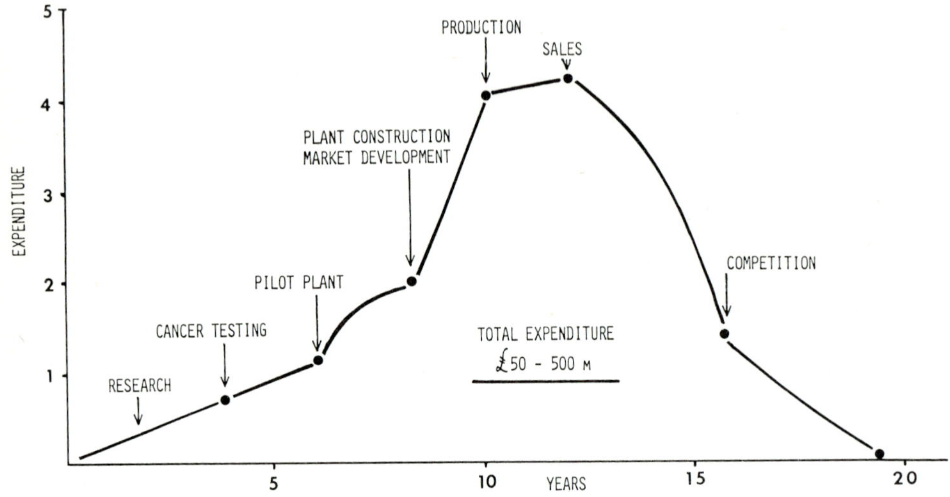

Figure 6.2 The cumulative costs of developing chemical products

cumulative costs incurred during this period. These variations can be between 10 and 20 years and between £50 million and £500 million. An average pharmaceutical, for example, probably reaches 'break-even' point between 10 and 12 years, and costs in the region of £50 million, whereas a large tonnage commodity chemical could reach ten times this cost figure in 15–20 years. At the other end of the scale, new dyestuffs based on minor chemical variation of established products might get into production for about £1 million.

The rate of expenditure varies according to capital outlay on pilot and main manufacturing plants, cost of production and sales and, at a later stage, on the further expenditure needed to meet competition on expiry of patents. Only when sales commence do the cumulative costs begin to fall, and only after the 'break-even' point is there a net gain to the company. The viability of the enterprise and the ability to finance new investment depend on the length of this period of 'profitability'. It rarely extends beyond two decades except where commodity chemicals are concerned. Such chemicals should, of course, receive most attention in determining possible carcinogenic hazards.

The introduction of new products is very variable, both in rate and scale, but we can assume that about forty *new* products reach the market-place each year in the UK. This does not include new formulations or minor variations of established products, but refers to products which are newly invented and, because little or nothing is known, need to be tested for their carcinogenicity in case of possible risk to worker or consumer. If we assume that one of these forty proves to be carcinogenic, then the costs incurred amount to £25·2 million (Table 6.2). Although this figure seems very large, it represents between

Table 6.2 Cost to industry (e.g. ICI Ltd)

Assume 40 new products per annum, of which all require testing and one is a carcinogen

Testing	0·5 × 40 = 20·0
Capital	5·0
Monitoring	0·2
	£25·2 m.

Total costs of production 40 × 50 = £2000 m.,

i.e. marginal cost of cancer testing = 1·26%

1·26% and 12·6% of the total cumulative costs of the forty projects (assuming that these lie between £50 million and £500 million per product) and it is this simplistic comparison of test costs and production costs which has resulted in the complacent assumption that the chemical industry can easily afford to be more safety-conscious, and indeed is verging on the criminally negligent if it is not.

The reality is very different. In the first place, these figures apply only if carcinogenicity testing is undertaken on chemicals destined for production, and then only when total costs over the 10–20-year span are considered. In fact, several thousand chemicals are evaluated and rejected before a likely candidate for production is identified. Many of those rejected will have been subjected to cancer testing, because the time required to test adequately demands that an early start be made if the evaluation is to be completed before a pilot plant is built. Current legislative trends indicate that such testing will increase; that is, many more chemicals will need to be subjected to cancer tests at an earlier stage in their development, in fact before many of the other problems governing successful development are solved. This trend will compound the second aspect of the problem, namely that it is not a question of the effect on total costs at all, but of the effect on cash flow at the research and development stage, for it is at this stage that the burden of testing falls and can be crippling.

If, for example, the R&D budget for a £50 million project is about £10 million over 5 years – and cancer testing at £0·5 million over 3 years costs £0·17 million per annum – cancer testing takes 8·5% of the R&D budget for those 3 years. A company like ICI Limited spends £100 million every year on R&D, and 8·5% of this represents a team of about 500 researchers. If such a team could produce only one new product per year, the financial consequences of not doing so, when discounted, will exceed £100 million over a 20-year period. If cancer testing has to be extended to many research chemicals (as might be the case if currently proposed legislation requires testing of all isolated chemicals, or chemicals produced in quantities of greater than 1 tonne per annum), the financial consequences are incalculable but certainly enormous; and probably more than the gross domestic budget could easily bear.

There are a number of ways by which the problem can be resolved but all demand recognition that one of the indispensable foundation-stones of an industrial society is a chemical industry which is not fettered by unreasonable and untutored concerns with safety. We must recognize that the industry is not the 'evil giant' to be slaughtered in the best fairy tale tradition, but a vital asset to be used sensibly in pursuit of wealth. In the first approach, extensive cancer testing should only be undertaken if a chemical is destined to go into production. This means that extensive testing need only be undertaken when the economics will allow it. There has to be, however, some protection of people working with development chemicals to ensure they are not exposed to potent carcinogens. It is possible that the short-term tests under development would suffice for this purpose. In order to be sure of this, however, the tests would need to undergo intense evaluation which would probably demand the combined efforts of industry, academics and governmental departments. This constitutes the second approach and such a task should take account of all of the information which allows a conclusion on possible carcinogenicity, such as chemical structure and relationship to known carcinogens. This must be an important part of any evaluation. Although there are many instances where the significance of chemical structure is not known, there are many where it is, and the aim must be to extend our understanding of this aspect to the extent that renders animal testing superfluous.

The third task will be to determine what kind of safeguards are necessary to enable a known carcinogen to be manufactured safely. Establishing such criteria would be, again, a task to be shared by industry and government.

It is conceivable that eventually the screening procedures could themselves

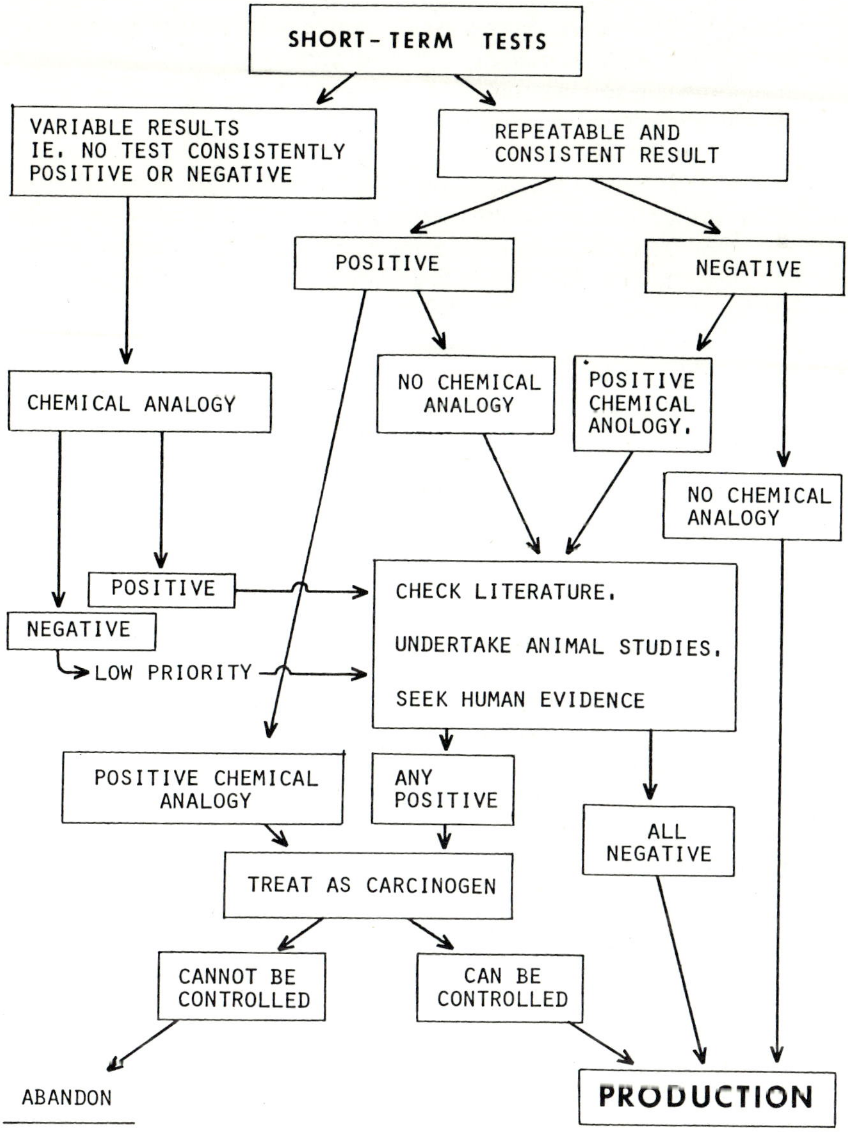

Figure 6.3 A decision scheme which might eventually allow the use of properly evaluated short-term tests to determine safety from cancer hazard in the work place

suffice to determine relative safety or otherwise of new chemicals. Such would be the case if the efficiency of prediction of carcinogenicity equalled that achievable by animal studies, or was so close that the chance of a false positive was small enough not to warrant the expense of animal studies.

These notions can be integrated into a decision-making scheme (Figure 6.3) towards which the combined efforts of industry, government and academics could work constructively together. Such a scheme indicates those topics (short-term tests, animal studies, industrial control) where more effort is needed before the scheme could be accepted; but it also provides for the essential learning process which we need to undergo in respect of chemical structure–function activity. The eventual adoption of such a scheme would certainly ease the cost burden on research and development, provided the range of chemicals tested is not extended.

We should not, of course, forget that carcinogenicity testing is now only one of the burdens which industry shoulders in its attempts to reach the market-place. Many other hazards loom in the minds of the untutored bureaucrat and it has become a kind of administrative game to construct schemes which ensure that no material with any conceivable hazard is ever put to use. Such schemes rarely include more than sketchy outlines of the cost to the communities they are intended to protect, and these are based on an economic illiteracy unrelated to the realities of cash flow. In the conclusions (below) the words 'cancer' and 'carcinogenesis' could be replaced by the term 'chronic toxicity' and be even more applicable to the immense tasks facing our chemical industry today.

CONCLUSIONS

1. Cancer testing should only be undertaken for chemicals destined to go into production, and should be regarded as a cost of production.
2. There should be industry-wide collaboration on the development of reliable short-term test procedures.
3. There should be industry/government collaboration on establishing the safeguards needed for a given potency of carcinogenesis.

Commentary

The effort and cost required for toxicity testing represent such a charge on our resources, particularly the scarcest resource of all – the innovative scientist – that there is definite slowing of original research into novel projects and even, in a self-defeating manner, into the mechanisms of carcinogenicity and tests for this property. The justification for the diversion of emphasis depends on society's view of what it wants and how much it is prepared to pay to satisfy its desires. Cancer is a particularly emotive subject, so public pressures to conduct more tests which, superficially at least, will protect humanity from exposure to cancer-producing agents, will be considerable.

Whether the entire financial cost of toxicity testing should be regarded as expenditure on R&D or on Production is more than just a neat point of accountancy. The apportionment influences thinking about the proportion of a firm's income available for innovative work, and it may result in inadvertent concealment or over-emphasis on such non-productive expenditure. Careful consideration should be given to every proposal for additional tests, to suspect materials. It is extremely difficult to conduct general screening of liability of safety testing with only too real an increase in cost or in the numbers of animals employed.

Within industry at large, particularly those parts where there may be widespread exposure to chemicals, growing concern with laboratory tests on compounds has been matched by interest in testing workers for effects of exposure to suspect materials. It is extremely difficult, to conduct general screening of large numbers of people, and there is no good evidence yet that it is useful, unlike detailed examination for specific lesions. It would be of general medical benefit to put some of the effort now expended on short-term tests for carcinogenic activity, and some of the large sums of money spent on long-term tests, into development of methods for assessing the effects on man of exposure to potentially hazardous chemicals. Perhaps cytogenetic analysis could be employed to demonstrate changes in the 'genetic apparatus' that would indicate hazardous exposure. Prevention of further exposure of the person might then save him from additional risk, if the detected change were to occur in the latent period before continued ingestion of the material led to onset of, say, a tumour.

7

Lifetime carcinogenic studies in rodents, viewed from the standpoint of experimental design: weaknesses and alternatives

D. Salsburg

In its most general form, the statistical or mathematical concept of experimental design requires that the expected outcome of an experiment can be described in terms of a mathematical model, and the design is dictated by the desire to estimate parameters of that model or to distinguish which of several forms of that model best fits reality. R. A. Fisher is a major contributor to the theory of experimental design (see Reference 1 for a discussion of his pioneering work), but the idea that an experiment's structure should be controlled by a preconceived mathematical model is much older; going back, at least, to Galileo.

Sometimes the mathematical model is so ingrained in the science that no one thinks to question it. For instance, experiments with radiolabelled tracers assume that the decay rate can be modelled as a first-order process, and all conclusions are derived within that model. At other times, the concepts underlying the experiment are quite vague and the mathematical model is hidden in language that is too imprecise to allow for clear conclusions. This happens often in clinical trials, where it is not clear whether the object of the trial is to locate a treatment-induced change in average patient response or a treatment-induced change in the number of patients who respond.

After examining the agricultural experiments of the late nineteenth and twentieth centuries, R. A. Fisher showed (References 2 and 3, for instance) that, without careful forethought about the mathematical model underlying the experiment, it was very easy to confound effects and reach conclusions that were misleading or even false. I would like to propose that the current state of carcinogenic testing is similar to the state of agricultural research in 1919, and that we need to step back and apply Fisher-like thinking, lest we find ourselves caught in a mire of confusion and questionable conclusions.

We can think of biological experiments as being controlled by the mathematical models to varying degrees. In the most open fashion, there are experiments in which one is hunting for information that will lead to the construction of a reasonable model. You isolate a biological system and attempt to control some stimuli or intake, then you measure various forms of activity or response. Many of the carcinogenic experiments of the 1940s and 1950s were done in this vein. But, such exploratory research rapidly reaches a point of diminishing returns. Careful examination of results, and even more careful thought about what happened, will usually produce a large number of competing models, all of which could account equally well for what was seen.

Good scientific procedure requires more careful control. In more careful experiments, we attempt to create a situation where the failure to observe something or a drastic change in a measure will allow us to eliminate one or more of the competing models of effect. This is the level to which Fisher rapidly moved agricultural experimentation in the 1920s. Such experiments can be thought of as occurring in a series. This is because a good experiment provides us with leads to other possible effects that can be investigated in the next experiment. In fact, it may be that the most important aspect of a well-designed experiment is learning how better to design the next experiment.

A good example of the use of a sequence of experiments to first derive and then investigate mathematical models are H. F. Blum's studies in carcinogenesis by ultraviolet light [4]. In his initial work, Blum probed with wavelengths at which protein and nucleic acid resonate, in order to be reasonably sure he was looking at the effects of single quanta of energy. The next few experiments sketched in the dose–response pattern. Observation of the living animals during these experiments led him to recognize that an important and measurable outcome of these experiments was the rate of growth of an observable tumour. He then projected several mathematical models to account for the growth he measured. One model allowed for a latent period before the clone of wild cells began, another assumed that the clone began with the first capture of a quantum of energy, etc. He was able to eliminate several of the competing models by designing experiments in which he interrupted the dosing in a carefully planned fashion. This, in turn, led to further refinements to his model to account for unexpected observations from these experiments.

As Blum did in ultraviolet light experiments, it should be possible to run a series of lifetime feeding experiments that will enable us to construct a reasonable set of mathematical models with which we will then be able to evaluate the carcinogenicity of a given compound. If we had such a model, we could design a lifetime feeding protocol that could be used over and over as a bioassay of the degree of carcinogenicity associated with different compounds.

This, in fact, is what the proponents of the lifetime feeding study propose to do with the current designs. They would use these designs as if the experiment were a definitive assay, a final arbitrator for compounds that are labelled possible carcinogens as a result of short-term studies, molecular structure, or toxicity. Is it possible to use the lifetime study, as it is now designed, for a bioassay? To answer this, let us look at what bioassay is in other fields. A full discussion of mathematical models available for bioassay experiments can be found in Finney [5].

In general, one can think of a bioassay as a rigid stereotyped procedure in which one provokes a measurable biological response with varying amounts of compound in order to characterize the 'activity' of that compound. That is, in the typical bioassay, one measures the biological response at several different doses or titration of the investigational compound. These values are then compared to a similar sequence of responses produced by a compound of known activity, or they are compared to a standard curve evolved from earlier experiments. The comparisons are made within the framework of a mathematical model whose structure has been established by prior experimentation. The result is a statement about the relative potency of the unknown compound, or a statement that the unknown mixture contains a certain amount of standard compound or has activity equivalent to a certain amount of standard compound. In addition to such purposes, all bioassays have thresholds. That is, there is a level of biological measurement below which the assay cannot distinguish the presence of the material or activity sought. The operating characteristics of a good bioassay are usually known, so it is possible to include that threshold of response as one of the parameters of the mathematical model.

Sometimes a bioassay is used primarily to detect the presence of activity above the level of that threshold. If the lifetime feeding study is a bioassay, this would seem to be its major purpose. We seek to detect the presence of a biological activity called carcinogenesis. If so, what is the well-defined mathematical model whose structure has been established by prior experimentation?

There is a model implicit in many of the statements of its proponents (see, for instance References 6 and 7 and the US Federal Register of Tuesday, October 4, 1977, pp. 54148–54247, in which the US Dept. of Labour proposed standards for identifying carcinogens in the work-place). This model has been made more explicit by Mantel and Schneiderman [8], among others. The model assumes that this is a well-defined end-point in a given animal – the

Table 7.1 The Mantel–Schneiderman model of carcinogenicity

$$\text{PROB}\ \{\text{an animal will be observed with tumour}\}$$

$$= f\begin{pmatrix}\text{inherent characteristic of the test compound,}\\ \text{dose}\\ \text{time of exposure}\end{pmatrix}$$

$f \approx$ 0 if the inherent characteristic is absent

Otherwise,

f increases as dose increases

f increases as time of exposure increases

observance of a tumour. The probability that an animal will be observed with a tumour is thought of as a function of:

1. an inherent characteristic of the compound at test;
2. the dose of the compound if it has that characteristic; and
3. the amount of time the animal is exposed to the compound, if it has that characteristic.

Those who propose *in utero* exposure will add a fourth dimension to the domain of that function:

4. the reduction of an animal's natural defences against cancer.

Since we are looking for an increase in the probability of an event, and since each animal can supply us with only a 'yes' or 'no' value, the model implies that there is a threshold of observation, in the sense that, with a given number of animals we can be reasonably sure of picking up an increase in probability only if it exceeds a certain amount. Figure 7.1 displays the curve of the number of animals we need in order to be 90% sure of finding at least one with tumour, plotted against the probability of tumour for a given dose of the carcinogen. For very low probabilities, we need an unreasonable number of animals. If the model is correct, we can increase the proportion of animals with tumour by increasing the dose and/or the time of exposure, and, hence, be able to detect the inherent characteristic of carcinogenesis with a smaller number of animals.

Unfortunately, the model does not fit reality. First of all, there is a considerable amount of background random noise. That is, animals that are not treated with the compound in question, but which are kept as controls, tend to have tumours, too. The pattern and frequency of such tumours changes with species, strain, location of trial, and even time of year (see References 9 and 10, for example). The bioassay must now detect an increase in probability

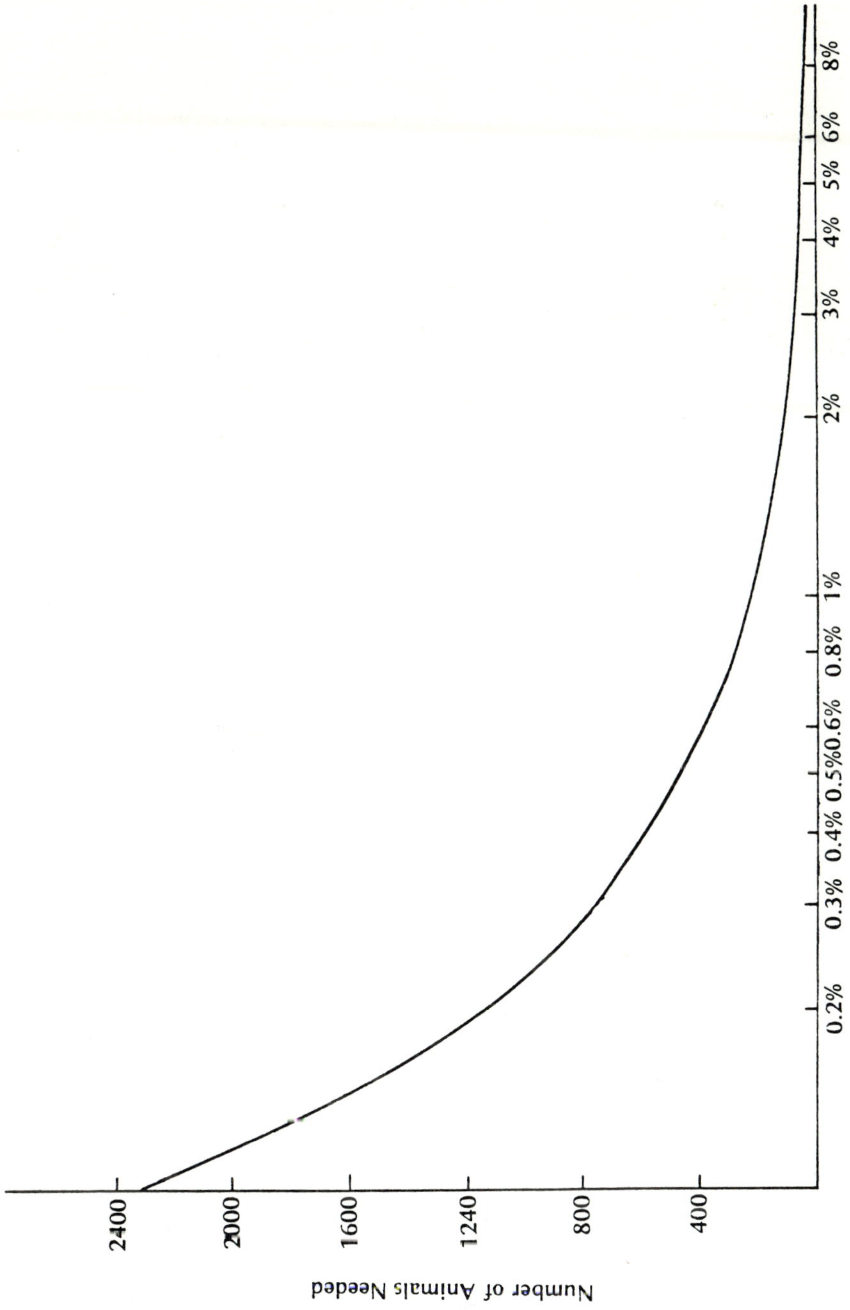

Figure 7.1 Number of animals needed to be 90% sure of having at least one animal with tumour, assuming no background incidence

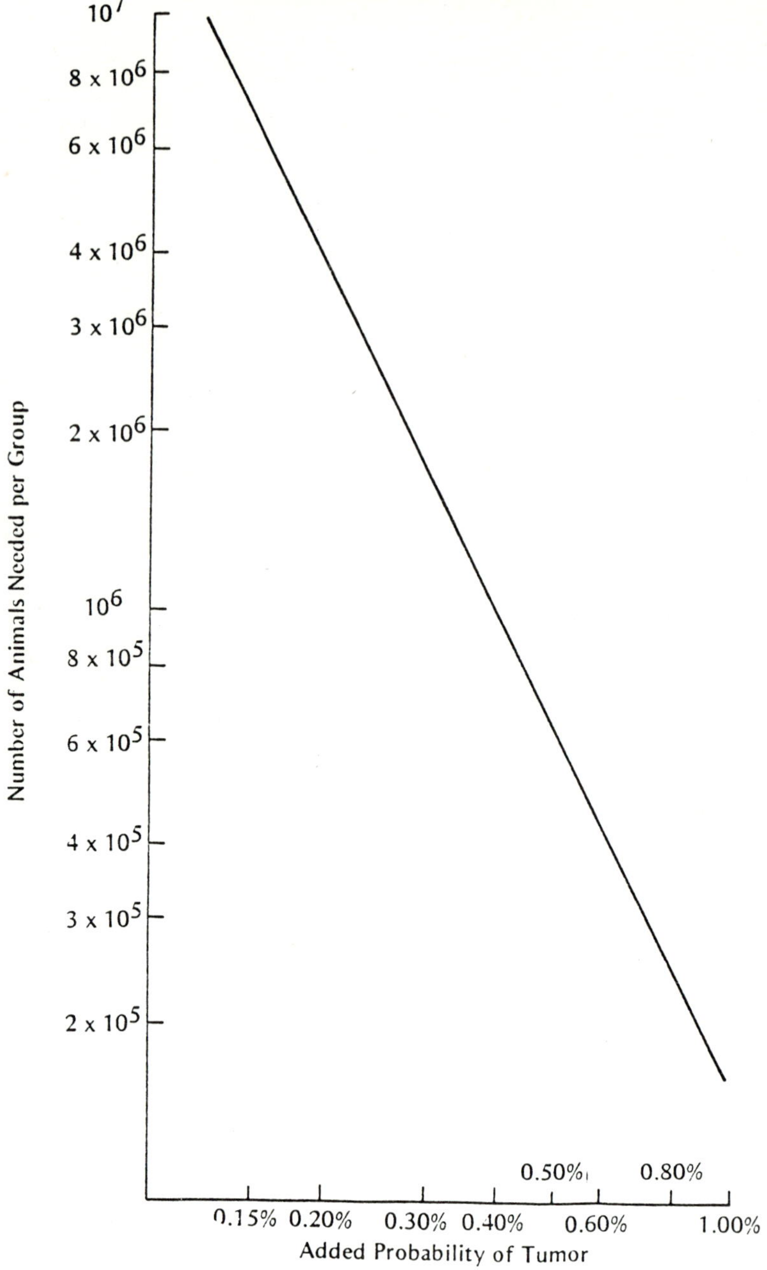

Figure 7.2 No. of animals needed per group to be 90% sure of detecting added probability of tumour when 10% of controls have tumours. $\alpha = 5\%$)

of tumour above that shown in the controls. The trade-off between number of animals and ability to detect a difference becomes more difficult. Figure 7.2 displays the curve for the number of animals versus difference in probability needed to be 90% sure of seeing such an effect, when 10% of the control animals tend also to have tumours.

As before, we can increase the sensitivity for a given number of animals if we can increase the difference in probability of tumour between the controls and treated. However, we can do this by extending the period of exposure only if extending exposure does not also increase the background rate to the same or a greater extent. If extending exposure increases the background rate, it could easily make detection even more difficult.

Proposals have also been made to modify the definition of what will be called a tumour-bearing animal (see Reference 7 for a discussion). This has led to arguments over whether one should consider only malignant tumours, all tumours, all hyperplastic lesions, or whether one should consider only gross tumours or the microscopic ones also. Many of these arguments seem to me to flow from a failure to think about them in terms of this mathematical model. From the standpoint of the model, it is clear that these techniques will increase the sensitivity only if they increase the difference in probability that an animal will be counted as tumour-bearing between controls and treated.

In order to know if extending exposure or modifying the definition of 'tumour-bearing animal' will increase the difference in probability, we will have to examine data from experiments already run, and probably construct a series of careful experiments that will further refine the mathematical model by allowing us to sketch in the algebraic form of this dose–time–definition-dependent probability function. My own analysis of data from lifetime studies has suggested to me that:

1. For both rats and mice, there is some point in time (about 18 months for the Sprague–Dawley rat) up to which there is a very low level of background noise and beyond which the number of control animals with tumours in certain organs increases very rapidly. If this is true, then the curves of tumour probability versus time of exposure may look like Figure 7.3. This has also been noticed by Nathan Mantel [11]
2. As we allow the definition of 'tumour-bearing animal' to include lesions that are not life-threatening or can be seen only in the microscope, we begin to have a large number of competing events, and can conceivably find out that a true carcinogen shows a lower probability of 'tumour' than the controls. I will return to this idea later.

The mathematical model has other errors in it to which I will also return later in the Chapter. For the moment, however, let us consider a bioassay based on that model in which we compare the proportion of tumour-bearing animals on various doses of compound to the proportion of tumour-bearing animals in the controls. One way to avoid some of the complications mentioned above is to restrict our attention to rare tumour types. We would then have an assay designed to discover compounds with a biological activity that induces an

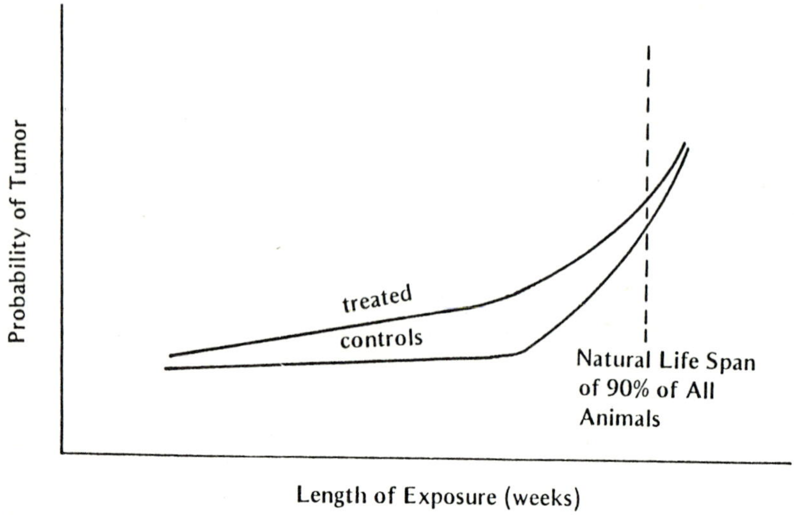

Figure 7.3 Hypothetical configuration of probability (tumour) versus length of study

animal to have a tumour in an organ not normally prone to tumour. In our mathematical model, the probability of such a tumour increases with increasing dose and with increasing time of exposure, but the probability of such a tumour in the controls remains relatively constant as we allow for increasing exposure time. We can now calculate the threshold of such an assay.

Figure 7.4 gives us the trade-off between number of animals per dose and increase in tumorigenesis, assuming that the control incidence is less than or equal to 0.1%. I have plotted this on log–log paper and shown the extreme end of the curve. Note that a direct consequence of the model is that, no matter how many animals are put on test, there remains an undetectable additional probability of tumour. If this model is correct, society is forced to make decisions. We must be willing to find a trade-off point. How much scientific resources will we expend for a given compound, and how fine-tuned a difference do we wish to detect? In a very simplistic view of that trade-off, to be 90% sure that a compound at test will not cause one cancer in a population of N people, we will have to test the compound on $0.02N^2$ animals per group. If N is 200 million people, the number of animals is more than 10^{14}

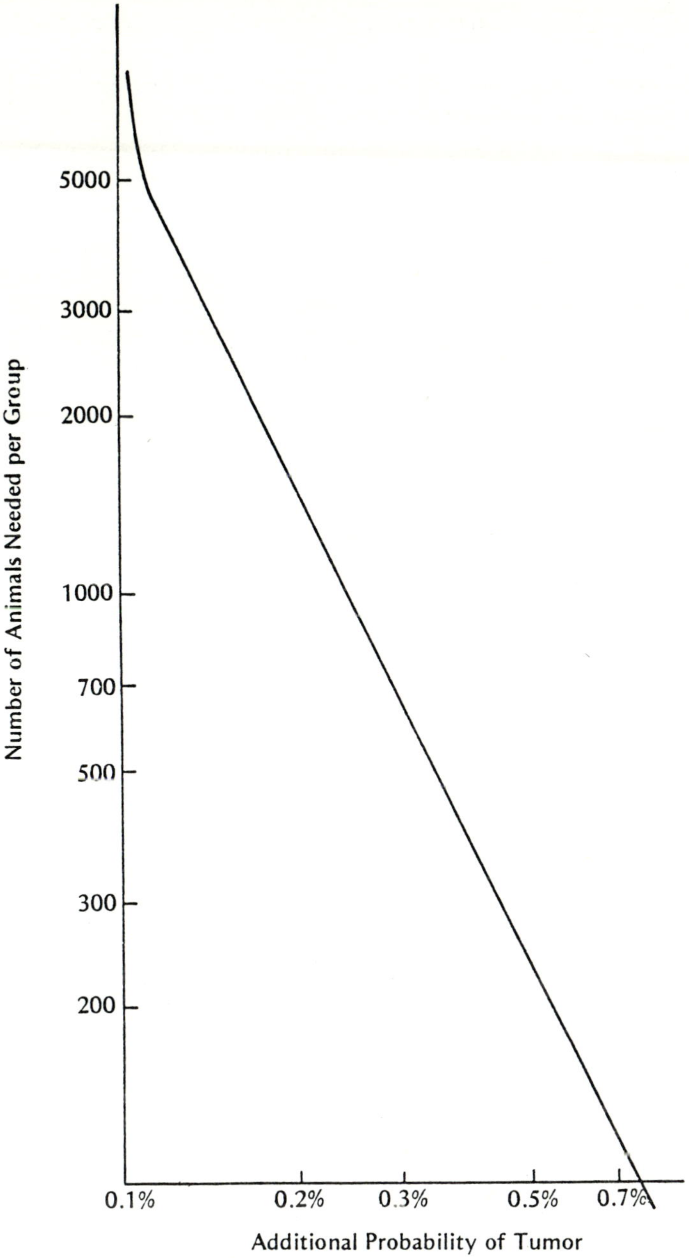

Figure 7.4 No. of animals needed per group to be 90% sure of detecting added probability of tumour when 0.1% of controls have tumours. $\alpha = 0.05$)

If the mathematical model is correct, then those involved in making regulatory decisions should have a clear understanding of this trade-off. Before we spend $200 000 or more on a carcinogenic study of a given compound, it is worth considering how much safety we are, in fact, buying.

Once we get beyond the compound which induces a rare tumour type, the mathematical model breaks down completely as a descriptor of reality. When we start looking at tumours that occur in 5% or more of the controls, we are faced with a mixed collection of events. The process of tumorigenesis and growth of cancer in a living animal is not fully understood, but we know enough about it to show that it cannot be modelled as a simple probability of a well-defined event occurring in a single animal. When we examine a dead animal we can find malignant tumours, gross tumours that are not malignant, and lumps and bumps that must be examined under the microscope to be sure what they are. The lumps and bumps might contain tissue with hyperplastic cells, or they might contain a clump of cells that appear to be malignant, or they might contain only non-tumorous inflammatory lesions. In addition, routine slices taken from certain organs might also reveal clumps of hyperplastic or neoplastic cells that could not be suspected from gross autopsy. There is a good reason to believe that, if allowed to live to an old age, there is a high probability that an animal will have such microscopic lesions, and a slightly smaller probability that it will have gross but non-life-threatening lesions. Autopsy reports [14] suggest that this is also true of the human. If we wish to model this process in order to detect the influence of a chemical compound on it, we are forced to the details of the carcinogenic process from at least three different standpoints:

1. We can think of a tumour starting from a single modified cell, then the clone has to reach about 10 000 cells before it can be observed grossly. Clones of smaller size will be found strictly by chance if we take a random slice of tissue and examine it under the microscope. Thus, the finding that an animal has a tumour falls into two phases. If the tumour is gross we can be fairly certain of finding it; but, if the tumour is microscopic, the probability that we will find it is a function of the way in which we sample the tissues of the animal. Suppose our sampling rule is that we take a standard slice of each of several organs plus a slice of all grossly observable lumps and bumps. Suppose, further, that in both the control and treated animals microscopic tumours can be found scattered with equal probability in a given tissue, but that one of the effects of the compound was to cause nodules of normal tissue to grow in that organ, or to induce cysts within the tissue. These nodules and cysts will be found and sampled, along with small bits of surrounding tissue, thus increasing the probability that a microscopic tumour will be found – even if the compound has had no effect on those tumours.

2. The compound might not have any effect on carcinogenesis, *per se*, but it might cause these microscopic tumours to grow more rapidly (as Blum discovered occurs with continual dosing of ultraviolet light) so that there are a larger number of gross tumours in the treated animals. Or, the compound might enhance the growth of one type of tumour leading to a higher occurrence of metastatic tumours. Both these events can be considered serious enough to indict the compound, but they are distinctly different from the concept of a carcinogen which causes an inheritable change in a single cell and starts an irrevocable process of cancer. The other effects could conceivably be strictly a phenomenom of the high doses used, and it might be possible to estimate a 'no-effect' dose.
3. For some tumour types, there is strong evidence that almost all control animals would come down with such a tumour if only they lived long enough. Test compounds could cause a decrease in the median time to such tumour. Or, by killing off enough 'weak' animals at the higher and toxic doses, they could increase the median time to what tumours are observed. Or they might produce a mixture of these two effects. The way in which such a compound 'causes' a change in median time to tumour may involve initial inheritable modifications of the cells or it may involve nothing more than a change in the general rate of metabolism for the entire animal. We may never be able to distinguish among different causes, but if we attempt to model this type of observation in terms of time-to-tumour, we shall have to include, in our model, measurements of the size and severity of the lesion, since tumours continue to grow in living animals beyond their initial appearance.

We can, of course, continue to use the simplistic mathematical model of tumorigenesis as a probability which is a function of dose and time, and apply this to the large variety of possible observations we get when we deal with tumour types that occur in the controls. If we do so, however, the assay is no longer specific. Instead, we will find ourselves on a hunting expedition where we are comparing all possible combinations of tumour types and sites.

Table 7.2, which has been presented elsewhere, shows what can happen with such a hunting expedition. If we examine the usual number of tissues in each animal and have three doses of compound compared to controls with 50 animals per sex per dose, we end up making more than 70 comparisons of control to treated. If we blindly apply 5% tests of statistical significance to these comparisons, this is how often we can be wrong and indict an innocent compound strictly by chance alone. These estimates are based upon a Monte Carlo study I ran using the incidence of commonly occurring tumours from long-term studies conducted at Pfizer.

It has been proposed that we can adjust the statistical tests to declare significance at the 1% level and reduce this false positive rate. However, we will still label many compounds as 'carcinogens' when the activity observed may be tumour-enhancement rather than true tumorigenesis. It may turn out that such tumour-enhancement is relatively common when we apply high doses of biologically active substances to rodents for their entire lifetimes. If so, we will soon find ourselves with a large catalogue of 'carcinogenic' compounds, without being able to distinguish between those that are dangerous at any dose and those that are tumour-enhancing only at exaggerated doses.

Table 7.2 Monte Carlo estimates of probability of a false positive (nominal alpha-level 5%)

Species	*Length of study* (months)	*No. Organs/*	*Percentage of false positives*
Male rats	24	5	51·2
Female rats	24	4	19·6
Male mice	18	5	21·5
Female mice	18	5	13·6
Male hamsters	19	3	12·1
Female hamsters	19	4	12·5
Male mice	20	5	57·3
Female mice	20	5	50·2

At the same time, we might miss some really bad compounds whose effect occurs early in the animal's life but are then swamped by similar events that occur in the controls just prior to sacrifice. If the effect is life-threatening, of course, we will see it in the early tumour-related deaths of the dosed animals. But one can conceive of a situation where the early tumours induce a higher level of clinical morbidity but not severe enough to bring about early sacrifices which might uncover the event.

If we are going to consider tumour types that occur in the controls and if we still wish to avoid either indicting 20–50% of all biologically active compounds (as appears to be happening now) or failing to catch the morbid but not mortal compound, then we will have to model the process with more complicated mathematics. From the more complicated mathematical model, we will then have to derive modified experimental designs. I have suggested a few such designs in Reference 13, but they are based on my own speculation about what might be useful mathematical models. What we need is more definitive knowledge. We need to move to the level of experimentation that Fisher imposed on agricultural research in the 1920s.

In particular, we need to construct a series of experiments whose design evolves as we evolve the models that best describe the process. Past experimentation in carcinogenesis has been aimed primarily at causing the process with a few well-studied compounds in order to understand how to cure it. We need experiments now which examine the relationship between the process of cancer and much broader classes of compounds, in order to understand how ingestion of toxic or near-toxic doses of chemicals influence that process. Some of these experiments can be relatively short-term. For instance, we will need to sketch in the effects on old-age lesions and can probably start with older animals; or we may want to look at the induction of microscopic tumours in animals in the prime of health. Some of these studies may have already been done, but have been buried in the vast flood of unco-ordinated experimentation that plagues the field of cancer research. But, in the end, we will need to conduct a series of well-designed lifetime experiments, with the 2–3-year delay involved in each one of them. If these experiments could be organized from a central planning body or bodies, the time needed to derive usable mathematical models might be shortened, but we are still talking in terms of years.

I have said 'we' need to design a sequence of good experiments to establish adequate mathematical models of the process. That 'we' will have to include teams of biologists, pathologists, and statisticians. For instance, the pathologists with whom I have worked believe that they can recognize the unusual patterns of morphology that enable them to distinguish between 'naturally' occurring tumours and those induced by test compounds, and that, as a result, there is little chance of missing a 'really bad actor'. Statisticians are experts in measurements. Surely the two disciplines ought to be able to combine, to produce a graded coding of pathology that will exploit that insight and give us far more informative measurements from each animal than a simple 'yes' or 'no' as is implied in the probability of tumour model. Good science requires the imaginative interplay of mathematical modelling and careful observation. Such an interplay has been missing in the past development of the lifetime feeding study and much confusion has been bred as a result.

So, where does that leave us? It appears to me that the lifetime feeding study is far from a 'definitive assay' for carcinogenesis. Unless we restrict it to the search for compounds which induce a rare tumour type, it lacks the elemental mathematical modelling that is needed for a bioassay. If we attempt to use it for more complicated situations, the current modelling is sufficient to make it hardly more than an open-ended search for cancer-related events. To mix metaphors, it is like looking for a needle in a haystack with a smoking torch. As much as I would like to find the needle of cancer causation, I fear we are in greater danger of burning down the haystack of chemical innovation or, at least, of being blinded by the smoke of our own confusion.

Let us step back and admit that it is premature to use this tool as a means of identifying chemical carcinogens among drugs and environmental and occupational hazards. Then let us launch a concerted effort to find out what this tool is capable of finding out for us and wherein it is capable of error.

References

1 Fisher, R. A. (1933). The contribution of Rothamsted to the development of the science of statistics. Annual Report. Rothamsted Experimental Station, pp. 45–50 (appears as paper No. 103 in *Collected Papers*, vol. 3)

2 Fisher, R. A. (1926). The arrangement of field experiments. *J. Minist. Agric.* (GB), **33,** 503 (Appears as paper No. 48 in the *Collected Papers of R. A. Fisher*, vol. 2, p. 83 (University of Adelaide Press, 1973)

3 Fisher, R. A. (1927). Studies in crop variation. IV, *J. Agric. Sci.* **17,** 548 (appears as paper No. 57 in the *Collected Papers*, vol. 2)

4 Blum, H.F. (1959). *Carcinogenesis by Ultraviolet Light; An Essay in Quantitative Biology* (Princeton: Princeton University Press)

5 Finney, D. J. (1952). *Statistical Methods in Bioassay*. (New York: Hafner)

6 Nelson, N. *et al.* (1971). FDA Advisory Committee on Protocols for Safety Evaluation: Panel on Carcinogenesis Report on Cancer Testing, *Toxicol. Appl. Pharmacol.*, **20,** 419

7 Shubik, P. *et al.* (1977). General criteria for assessing evidence for carcinogenicity of chemical substances: Report of the Subcommittee on Environmental Carcinogenesis, National Cancer Advisory Board, *J. Natl. Cancer Inst.*, **58,** 461

8 Mantel, N. and Schneiderman, M. (1975). Estimating 'safe' levels, a hazardous undertaking. *Cancer Res.*, **35,** 1379

9 MacKenzie, W. *et al.* (1972). Comparisons of neoplasms in six sources of rats. *J. Natl Cancer Inst.*, **50,** 1243

10 Sher, S. (1972). Mammary tumours in control rats; literature tabulation. *Toxical. Appl. Pharmacol.*, **22,** 562

11 Mantel, N. (1977). Affidavit presented to the Hearing Clerk of the Food and Drug Administration, U S DHEW, in the matter of actions and procedures for evaluating assays of carcinogenic residues in edible products in animals (March 21)

12 Shubik, P. and Hartwell, J. (1969). *Survey of Compounds Which Have Been Tested for Carcinogenic Activity*, PHS Publication No. 149, US Govt Printing Office (subsequent volumes were prepared on contract with the NCI and bring the survey up to 1975)

13 Salsburg, D. (1977). The use of statistics when examining lifetime studies in rodents to detect carcinogenicity, *J. Tox. Environ. Health.* **2,** 613

14 Huyoshi, Y. *et al.* (1977). Malignant neoplasms found by autopsy in Hisayama, Japan during the first ten years of a community study, *J. Natl Cancer Inst.*, **59,** 13

Commentary

The probability model of animal carcinogenicity testing carries several unpalatable implications. Perhaps the worst is the fact that the statistical power of the test can only distinguish a marked effect, i.e. approximately a 3- or 4-fold increase above the background incidence of neoplasms. Even an increase in the numbers of animals in each dose-group results in relatively little improvement, at least not unless an unimaginably and unmanageably large number were used.

It is important, too, that the background incidence of tumours in untreated or control animals be kept as low as possible. The reason for this is implicit in the method of statistical analysis used to analyse the results. If the spontaneous incidence of neoplasms is high the variance also rises and the result of the experiment will become lost in the background noise. In mathematical terms we are concerned in the probability model with the variance of a binomial. The variance is a linear function of the probability at low levels of uncertainty, i.e. the power of the test to distinguish between two possibilities is high. But if the variance is greater than about 5%, it is no longer linearly related to the mean, and instead it rises as the quadratic of the uncertainty. The result is very rapid loss of the power of a test to differentiate a carcinogen from an inactive compound.

Short-term mutation tests may be viewed more simply in this context, because there is a direct relationship between the action of a compound and the observed effect. In an animal test, on the other hand, the link between administration of a chemical and appearance of tumours at various sites, or sooner than in controls, is so indirect that there is no assurance that these effects are events with a well-defined probability characteristic.

There is much interest in the effects of diet on carcinogenesis. The claimed activities range from enhancement of neoplasia by increase in total fat and unsaturated fatty acids to prevention by a reduced amount of protein. Confounding these views is the suggestion that most, if not all, apparently spontaneous carcinogenesis is really due to contamination of the diet by various oncogenic mycotoxins or substances with potent oestrogenic activity. The interrelationships between these conflicting influences, the activity of the substance being investigated and its effect on the nutrition of the animals is so complex that, as one speaker said, 'We can seek only for confused enlightenment'.

This is the mathematical view, and it has been attacked on biological grounds by the unsupported assertion that, if the animals employed have a low incidence of tumours, it is because they are innately 'resistant' to carcinogenesis, and are probably unable to respond to carcinogenic chemicals and should not be used to test for this property.

8

Problems facing the regulatory authorities

I: Problems with medicinal products

G. Jones

The following remarks apply only to the problems involved in regulating drugs or medicinal products. The manufacture and supply of medicinal products is now strictly and comprehensively controlled by legislation. Although legislation involving medicines can be traced back to the sixteenth century the major legislation controlling drugs is the Medicines Act of 1968 which was the final outcome, in the UK, of the thalidomide tragedy. The Act provides for the establishment of a licensing authority, consisting of the health and agriculture ministers, which grants clinical trial certificates (CTC) to permit clinical trials and product licences (PL) to permit marketing. Applications for certificates or licences are submitted in the first instance to Medicines Division of the Department of Health and Social Security (DHSS). These applications are assessed by the licensing authority on the basis of quality, safety and efficacy. In this assessment the licensing authority is assisted by the professional staff of the division and various advisory committees of experts set up under the act. The most well known of these committees is the Committee on Safety of Medicines (CSM) which gives advice on the majority of applications for new medicines; it is itself assisted by a variety of sub-committees. Other committees have also been set up in the past two years; viz. the Committee on Review of Medicines (CRM) which is concerned with reviewing licences of existing products, particularly those on the market before the Medicines Act came into force, and the Committee on Dental and Surgical Materials (CDSM) which assesses, as its name implies, applications for products outside the main provisions of the Act.

Ordinarily applications which are minor and straightforward or variations on existing licences are assessed by the professional staff of the division, and if all is well a clinical trial certificate or product licence will be granted by the licensing authority. If the application concerns a major new drug, or if there are any problems, then it is referred to the CSM (or CDSM as the case may be). This referral is mandatory, under the Act, if the licensing authority intends to refuse the application. Preparation of applications is the responsibility of the manufacturer. Detailed guidelines for the preparation of applications are issued by the Department, and revised from time to time. Applicants who are refused the grant of a CTC or PL have the right to make representations to the CSM in the first instance and secondarily to the Medicines Commission. The latter body, which is often confused with the CSM, is also established under the Act but has a broader composition than the CSM. In addition to the role indicated above it also provides advice of a general nature on medicines.

Apart from the routine work of processing CTC and PL applications the licensing authority also has to deal with problems resulting from the assessment of new evidence on the safety or efficacy of marketed products. These problems can occur at any time and are usually referred to the CSM for advice.

All of the bodies referred to above are involved in the problems relating to carcinogenicity. But in practice decisions of the licensing authority are largely determined by advice from the professional staff of Medicines Division, the CSM and one of the Sub-Committees (the Sub-Committee on Toxicity, Clinical Trials and Therapeutic Efficacy). The problems of carcinogenicity testing can be discussed under the following headings:

CARCINOGENICITY TESTING REQUIREMENTS

The major questions are: which compounds should be tested, how should testing be conducted and when should testing be conducted? The licensing authority and its various advisory committees have been concerned with these questions for some time. About a year ago, because of the difficulties involved in making decisions on CTC and PL applications, a working party was set up to examine these problems. This working party consisted of members of the CSM and its Sub-Committees and scientific experts from the pharmaceutical industry. The final report of this working party is currently being considered by all the interested parties. The consultative document makes the following points:

Which compounds should be tested?

Compounds will require testing if they fall into either of two broad groups.

First, testing will be required on all products which are intended for long-term use or frequent intermittent use or which are retained (or their metabolites) in the body for a long time. Secondly, products will require testing if there is a high index of suspicion due to their chemical structure (i.e. relationship to known carcinogens) or biological activity (e.g. adverse effects on fertility or embryogenesis, or proliferative changes in various issues). Difficulties often arise in practice in interpreting these guidelines, e.g. in determining the degree of structural similarity between a known carcinogen and a new product, or in assessing the nature of proliferative changes.

How should testing be conducted?

Carcinogenicity testing will involve *in vivo* studies in animals. Studies should normally be conducted in two species, with drug administration at three dose-levels. It is desirable that metabolism of the drug in the chosen species should be similar to that in man, although it is recognized that in practice testing will nearly always involve rodents (mouse, hamster and rat). Drug administration should be by the proposed route of administration in man, and should be conducted for 18 months in the mouse and hamster, and 2 years in the rat. Because of the length and difficulty of the study animal husbandry of the highest quality is necessary. Also terminal autopsies and histopathology should be of the highest standard. Professional statistical advice on the design of the study, and analysis of the results, should be obtained.

When should testing be conducted?

In all cases testing should be completed and assessed before compounds are marketed. Where drugs are intended for long-term use it will usually be necessary to complete testing before the drug is used on a long-term basis, even if the latter occurs during clinical trials. Where the carcinogenic risk is due to chemical structure or biological activity it will usually be necessary to complete testing before any clinical trials commence.

Not all the points mentioned above have been adopted yet, nor has it been decided when any new guidelines will become operative. At the moment, for example, it is not mandatory to conduct carcinogenicity testing on compounds intended for long-term use, although the UK is signatory to an EEC agreement which states that testing under such circumstances may be required. Other points mentioned above, however, on the conduct of testing and the time of testing, are already accepted by the CSM and have been applied to a variety of products; e.g. parenteral iron preparations, -blocking agents, oestrogen/progestogen combinations. In some cases it is difficult to state in advance precisely which requirements will apply to individual products. A flexible approach to the interpretation of guidelines is therefore essential.

INTERPRETATION OF DATA

The major question is: on the basis of the evidence available does this compound present a carcinogenic risk to animals and/or man? In the first instance attention must be paid to the source of the evidence. Although most of the data in this field are obtained in animal experiments sometimes results are available in man. Since it is accepted that, other factors being equal, data derived from human use transcend in quality data from any other source, one can classify the source of evidence in decreasing order of quality as follows:

Human data

Epidemiological evidence to man, although rarely available and usually retrospective, provides the strongest evidence. There are many difficulties in interpreting retrospective studies due to the selection of controls, but the great advantage is that one can analyse data from the most relevant species exposed to normal clinical usage of the drug. One should not scorn even occasional case reports since these are particularly valuable for very rare tumours.

Animal tests

These represent the major source of data for assessment of carcinogenicity of drugs, either at CTC or PL stages of development. There is still debate regarding the value of testing medicinal products in rodents, particularly at doses which are often high multiples of the human therapeutic dose. Reservations have been expressed by the scientific community and by members of the general public who are concerned, quite properly, with the use of large numbers of animals for these purposes. Clearly there are dangers in extrapolating results from animals to man because of differences in drug metabolism, species responses, etc., but two points should be borne in mind. Firstly, nearly all human carcinogens can be shown to be carcinogenic in animal tests conducted along the lines described above (the converse of course is not true). Secondly, most products, when tested in this way, product negative results unless there is some structural relationship to a known carcinogen.

Screening tests for carcinogenicity

In practice these involve mutagenicity or transformation assays. Although there is a correlation between these tests and formal *in vivo* testing, the incidence of false positives and false negatives with short-term assays is too high to regard them as satisfactory replacements. These tests are not mandatory for drugs at the moment. If such tests have been conducted, and produce positive results, then it is almost certain that the licensing authority would require complete testing *in vivo*. A negative result would not preclude the need for *in vivo* testing if the latter were judged necessary on the grounds referred to previously. Despite these reservations it is desirable that short-term screening tests are conducted on all drugs, for two reasons. First, if they turn out to be positive, they provide a good clue to the value of further commercial development of the compound; secondly, as the number of compounds tested increases, our knowledge and understanding of their value will also increase.

Apart from the source of the data any interpretation will take into account the quality of the data and the nature of the results. One assumes that the study is well designed and executed with considerable care. Because of the large numbers of animals used in a carcinogenicity test (usually 500 animals for each species) it is quite easy for errors to occur. High-quality animal husbandry and considerable attention to the details of dosing are therefore essential. Equally important are the conduct of histopathology and statistical analysis. In assessing the results the critical features are the numbers of benign/malignant tumours for each tissue in the dosed and control animals.

A raised incidence of malignant tumours is usually interpreted as posing a greater carcinogenic hazard than a similar increase in benign tumours. Other features influencing the degree of carcinogenic risk are mentioned below.

DECISIONS INVOLVING RISK–BENEFIT ASSESSMENT

The assessment or evaluation of risk and benefit are major areas of controversy. In practice, decisions have to be taken under two differing sets of circumstances.

(a) At the time of application of CTC or PL. In the case of CTC applications a decision has to be taken whether to permit trials or to place certain restrictions on the proposed trials. In the case of PL applications a decision has to be taken initially on whether the drug should be marketed and, if so, whether any form of warning is appropriate or whether use of the drug should be restricted to certain clinical indications.

(b) In the case of compounds already on the market, when new evidence comes to light, a decision has to be taken concerning revocation or variation of the licence.

Assessments of risk–benefit ratios in these two situations are different. If a product is already on the market one has to assume that patients are deriving benefit from the drug and revocation of the licence will deprive them of this benefit. Also withdrawal from the market of products with which the public is very familiar can produce a fair degree of alarm. However, in the case of products which are being assessed for the grant of a CTC or PL, the therapeutic benefit is potential rather than actual. Thus the 'burden of proof' rests more heavily on the licensing authority when decisions are taken on marketed products compared with drugs under development. Revocation of a licence or withdrawal of a CTC are all-or-nothing decisions. Variation, however, allows a graded response to any potential hazard. A licence may be varied to remove certain clinical indications or to require that a warning be included on the data sheet.

Decisions always involve an assessment of the risk and the benefit of the product in question.

EVALUATION OF RISK

This requires assessment of the source of evidence (epidemiological, animal studies, screening tests), quality of the data (design, controls, analysis) and nature of the results (benign/malignant tumours, dose-levels, etc).

The most frequent situation would involve results of animal studies, well designed and well conducted, indicating a raised incidence of malignant tumours in one tissue at doses several times higher than the human therapeutic dose. Although extrapolation of results from rodents to man is always open to question the current position is that compounds which are carcinogenic in animals are assumed to be potentially carcinogenic in man until the contrary can be established. A more precise assessment of the carcinogenic risk to man would depend on the proposed duration of clinical use, the dose-levels at which tumours appeared in animals, the latency of tumour appearance (if this can be estimated) and the frequency and nature of the tumours.

It would be fair to say that in most cases where clear positive results are obtained in animal tests, particularly for drugs in the development stage, the drug has no future. Many pharmaceutical companies voluntarily terminate development of the drug in advance of any decision by the licensing authority. Where results are not so clear or where the drug may offer considerable benefit then careful evaluation will be necessary.

One final point to be borne in mind is that the evaluation of risk is aimed at determining the degree of risk to an individual patient receiving the drug. The risk is independent of the numbers of patients receiving the drug; the latter determines the cost to society of any adverse event.

EVALUATION OF BENEFIT

For all drugs this requires, quite simply, an assessment of the efficacy of the product in reducing the morbidity or mortality associated with the disease in question. This will depend on the results of clinical trials comparing the product with placebo or other active agents. Assessment of the benefit of the drug will almost always involve a consideration of the efficacy of alternative drugs, if these are available, or even alternative techniques of therapy, e.g. surgery.

EVALUATION OF RISK IN RELATION TO BENEFIT

Evaluation of this nature always involves the exercise of judgment and cannot be quantified in mathematical terms since it involves several value-judgments. The reduction of risk–benefit assessment to numerical ratios of monetary values based on actuarial analyses of life-time earnings or legal compensation cases is not practised by the licensing authority or CSM. Each assessment involves unique factors, and different standards apply to different products. For example much higher degrees of carcinogenic risk are tolerated for all products intended for use in advanced malignant disease, whereas higher standards of safety prevail in the assessment of hypnotics. The evaluation of risk and benefit with respect to carcinogenicity is therefore no different in principle from similar judgments on the safety and efficacy of all medicinal products.

In the assessment of risk–benefit, with respect to carcinogenicity or safety and efficacy in general, no account is taken of social costs or cost–benefit analyses involving consideration of commercial or economic factors. Although such considerations are involved in policy formulation in other divisions of the DHSS (in relation to resource allocation) this approach has not been used in medicines division, for two reasons. Firstly, neither the CSM nor its professional staff are experts at economic analysis. Secondly, it has not been necessary, to date, to perform analyses involving these other factors since alternative products are usually available. However, one can visualize situations where such analyses might prove necessary, e.g. in the assessment of drugs for rare diseases.

Finally one must bear in mind that decisions often have to be taken in advance of precise knowledge. For example, in the case of progestogens there is considerable debate regarding the value of carcinogenicity testing in the beagle. A complete solution to this problem will probably require many years of further research. In the meantime the knowledge that two groups of progestogens can be distinguished on the basis of carcinogenicity results in beagles requires an immediate decision. In the USA testing in beagles has already been made an absolute requirement by the FDA. The current position in the UK is that, unless there are compelling reasons to do otherwise, progestogens should be tested in the beagle before marketing.

The views expressed in this Chapter are the responsibility of the author and do not represent the official views of the Department of Health and Social Security or the Committee on Safety of Medicines.

9

Problems facing the regulatory authorities

II: Problems in interpreting and implementing results from carcinogenicity studies

E. M. B. Smith

The Department of Health and Social Security (DHSS) has the responsibility for advising government on matters relating to carcinogenesis and examining human health hazard resulting from exposure to carcinogens.

The number of known human carcinogens is relatively small, and is in the region of thirty. The International Agency for Research on Cancer has identified, on the basis of strong evidence, approximately 150 substances which are carcinogenic in animals. The US National Institute of Occupational Safety and Health currently lists, on the basis of animal evidence of varying quality, no less than 2415 suspected carcinogens. Any substance producing an increased incidence of neoplasms in experimental animals may have a carcinogenic potential for man, and the uncertainty in purely numerical terms is a problem when assessing and evaluating possible human health hazard in this field.

Human carcinogens are usually identified epidemiologically, and this tends to be a retrospective process; whereas the prime task of regulatory authorities is ideally to ensure that man is not exposed to carcinogens.

There are many problems in the interpretation and evaluation of the results of carcinogenicity studies in animals, their extrapolation to man, and the assessment of risk and hazard. The terms risk and hazard are used interchangeably but perhaps they could be differentiated by regarding risk as a probability, which can be expressed in mathematical terms, whereas hazard can be considered as a more general concept embracing risk and other factors such as exposure. A chemical intermediate which occurs only transiently in an enclosed process can pose a carcinogenic risk but not present a significant hazard.

If animal studies were capable of straight extrapolation to man, decision-making and appropriate regulation would be relatively simple, always allowing for the inherent complexities of the legal process. It is easy to see that in the case of a substance which is a human carcinogen, which is man-made, has no practical uses and is not pleasurable or 'habit-forming', a complete ban on production would be fully justified and acceptable to all. However, things are not that simple, and the idea that all carcinogens are man-made and that their prohibition is an easy matter and would obviate all carcinogenic risk is clearly ill-founded. There are environmental carcinogens of significance for man which occur naturally (for example arsenic, chromates and asbestos), and the sun is a major cause of skin cancer. There are also carcinogens produced by plants, for example, aflatoxins, cycasin and safroles. The burning of hydrocarbon fuels, which is regarded as a very normal activity, gives rise to known carcinogens. The elimination of all carcinogens is not possible and, until the knowledge of mechanisms of carcinogenicity has reached a stage where the activity of carcinogens can be blocked or otherwise inhibited, practicable methods of protection for man will depend largely on the limitation, rather than on the abolition, of exposure. Control of carcinogens is a very complex issue with the ultimate form of control, namely total prohibition, possible in very few cases.

The object of a system of control is to reduce inevitable exposure to a safe level. Safety can be considered in an absolute sense, that is the complete absence of risk, but in practical terms it is a relative concept implying no detectable risk or increase in hazard. Because the perception of risk and evaluation of hazard are not absolute, judgments in this area are subjective. To quantify risks in the field of carcinogenesis presents formidable obstacles, and attempts to extrapolate directly from an order-of-risk determined in animal studies to a risk-for-man lack scientific validation. The same element of subjectivity applies also to benefits and thus to all risk–benefit considerations.

Mechanisms for generating and transmitting advice on carcinogenicity and carcinogenic risk exist in the DHSS, which has appropriately qualified permanent staff and an expert committee structure. The expert committee dealing with carcinogenesis forms part of the COMA structure. COMA is the abbreviation for the Committee on Medical Aspects of Chemicals in Food, Consumer Products, and the Environment. The Co-ordinating Committee and the associated expert committees on Toxicity, Carcinogenicity, Mutagenicity, and Physical Environment operate on the basis of referrals or requests for advice from a wide variety of sources; mainly, but not exclusively, government departments. Referrals to the Carcinogenesis Committee are usually for a decision on whether a substance should be considered a human carcinogen or poses a carcinogenic risk for man, and the Committee is also concerned with examining the relevance of advances in its scientific field of expertise and in preparing guidelines for carcinogenicity testing. These Guidelines, at present in draft form, are intended to provide general advice to those carrying out carcinogenicity studies in animals. In the case of a referral the Committee reviews and assesses data on chemical properties, animal studies, metabolic activity and human epidemiology, and gives its advice in the form of an opinion or a recommendation. Any legislative and regulatory actions are then the responsibility of the government departments concerned. For example, matters related to a possible carcinogenic risk in food will be dealt with by the Ministry of Agriculture, Fisheries and Food (MAFF) and the Food Additives and Contaminants Committee (FACC); a carcinogen in a consumer product by the Department of Prices and Consumer Protection (DPCP); and an environmental carcinogen by the Department of the Environment (DOE). The Health and Safety Executive (HSE) is charged with the control of carcinogens in the occupational environment, and can prohibit or define conditions under which substances considered to be established or suspected human carcinogens can be used in industry. The HSE has access to its own toxicological advice, including questions of carcinogenicity, but can refer for advice to the COMA expert committees. Similarly the voluntary Pesticides Safety Precautions Scheme, which has expertise in the field of carcinogenesis in its Scientific Sub-Committee, can also refer to COMA for advice.

The identification of animal carcinogens by means of experimental animal studies is accepted, as is that of human carcinogens by epidemiological methods. The results of short-term screening tests for carcinogenesis are seen as useful indicators in making decisions on full animal studies but not as replacements for them. There are difficulties in interpreting the results of animal studies. Where the results are not clear-cut, or where deficiencies in the methodology or in the actual conduct of the studies are apparent, a reasonable evaluation is not possible; it may then be necessary to defer decisions until more information is available. Problems of a practical significance arise where there is reasonable animal evidence of carcinogenicity but human epidemiology does not show an effect.

As each case is judged on the basis of the available evidence, with the inherent variations in sensitivity of the different approaches to testing, the nature and strength of recommendations to government departments can vary. Having made the basic decision that a substance does constitute a carcinogenic risk to man, further consideration must be given to reviewing the nature of the exposure and the numbers likely to be exposed, and also to any benefits.

The system for providing advice on carcinogenesis to government is certainly not static and is, in fact, currently undergoing an 'evolutionary' spurt to meet the demands of an increasing awareness of the problem of carcinogenesis and the demands for the protection of the population. Regulatory bodies must have balanced advice indicating the nature and extent of the hazard, the benefits, and those social and economic factors which assume considerable importance when firm decisions must be made.

The task of the DHSS, its expert advisers and the other governmental bodies involved is to identify existing carcinogens, assess their significance for man and devise methods for their control; as a corollary, reliable methods of prediction from the results of animal studies must be developed to ensure that new carcinogens are not introduced. While these methods are being developed the lack of certainty in predictive capability warrants the monitoring, wherever possible, of groups exposed to new chemicals. The DHSS has a key role to play in integrating the flow of information on carcinogenesis coming from laboratory studies, epidemiological field research, occupational exposure, and monitoring of morbidity in the general population.

Commentary

The UK Medicines Act (1968) states that the decision to permit or to refuse permission for a new medicine to be used in man should be based on considerations of safety and efficacy, but not solely of efficacy relative to other compounds of the same therapeutic type. Looked at in this way a regulatory authority has a particularly difficult task when it asked to decide about a new compound, which is a member of a group of which several other members are already available.

The present official attitude is that such a problem cannot involve entirely separate assessment of efficacy. A novel compound would have to be at least as efficacious and as safe as existing medicines for marketing permission to be granted. This is different from the first occasion when a new substance with an entirely novel action is to be considered. The decision here must involve a more difficult analysis of risk and benefit, without the guidance of prior experience of substances with the particular type of action.

An example of the results of such considerations is provided by the opinion of the UK Committee on the Safety of Medicines (CSM) about beta-blockers. Many compounds of this type have been marketed, and there is no evidence that any are carcinogenic in man. However, some drugs in this class have apparently caused tumours in animals. As a result, the CSM has stated that no clinical work with a new beta-blocker will be permitted unless animal tests have shown that it does not have a carcinogenic action. Their argument involves an element of comparison, because it is based on the free availability of other beta-blockers. The converse view would be advanced if a new class of drug was being introduced; namely that assessment would depend much more strictly on analysis of the likely benefits and risks of the new material.

10

The tetrazolium test for skin carcinogenicity

O. H. Iversen

The tetrazolium test was introduced by Iversen in 1962 for substances that were carcinogenic for the skin after topical application.

It is based on the fact that the colourless salt triphenyltetrazolium chloride is reduced to red formazan by the activity of the energy-generating processes in the mitochondria. If cells are not severely injured, and if the dose of tetrazolium reaching the cells is sufficient, but not toxic, the formazan deposition is proportionate to the oxygen consumption of the cells (Iversen, 1962). In injured cells, however, there may be blocks at different stages in the respiratory chain leading to an increase in the amount of formazan deposited. If cell membranes are injured, there may be an increased access of tetrazolium to the actual site of enzymes in the mitochondria, a condition which may also lead to increased deposition of formazan. In such cases the amount of formazan deposited is not proportionate to oxygen consumption. This is probably the basis for the tetrazolium test for skin carcinogens.

There are great biological variations between individual mice as regards the amount of formazan deposited in the epidermis under normal conditions. To counteract this, we painted one area of the back skin of hairless mice with the substance to be tested, and the control area was taken from another part of the same animal.

A study of early carcinogenesis with this method revealed (Figure 10.1) that after the application of a particular dose of the carcinogen tested, the amount of formazan deposited increased considerably during the first 1–3 days, and then was markedly reduced for many days. Non-carcinogenic skin irritants showed another pattern, with an immediate small reduction in the formazan deposition for several days, followed by a return to normal.

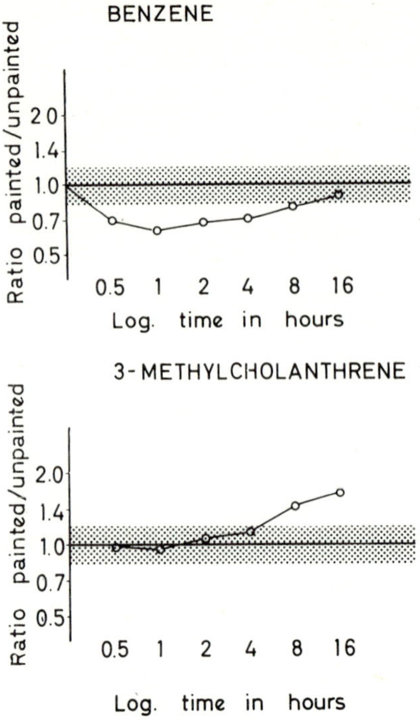

Figure 10.1 The deposition of formazan per mg dry epidermis at different time points after topical application to the skin of hairless mice

The increased formazan deposition seemed to be specific to the skin carcinogens, and when the test was repeated by Ben and Valentini in 1965, they got exactly the same results. When a carcinogen was tested, the ratio treated/untreated of formazan deposited per mg epidermis one day after application was always 1·20 or higher.

The dose is important. As shown in Table 10.1, 20-methylcholanthrene (MCA) gives no positive reaction until a dose of about 10 μg is applied. MCA is a strong carcinogen and a weak skin irritant.

Cantharidine, on the other hand, is a strong skin irritant and a very weak carcinogen. Table 10.2 shows the results obtained with different doses of cantharidine in benzene, and it is evident that strong doses of toxic substances kill cells completely, and then the formazan deposition is greatly reduced.

Thus, the tetrazolium method requires a relatively strong, but non-ulcerative dose of the substance.

One must keep in mind that most carcinogens show organ-specificity, and that for a proper test the tetrazolium method has to be applied to each individual organ. At our institute we are at present working with slices of liver

Table 10.1 Tetrazolium test with different doses of 3-methylcholanthrene

Amount applied (μg)	*Percentage solution in benzene*	*No. of mice*	*Test result*
0·4	1/128	16	0·898
0·8	1/64	16	0·792
1·6	1/32	16	0·818
3·1	1/16	32	1·107
6·3	1/8	32	1·168
25·0	1/2	32	1·361
50·0	1/1	16	1·410

Table 10.2 Tetrazolium test with different doses of cantharidine

Percentage solution in benzene	*No. of mice*	*Test result*
0·02	16	1·25
0·04	16	1·48
0·35	16	0·87

tissue after intraperitoneal injection of carcinogenic and non-carcinogenic substances, and the preliminary results are promising. Similarly, if the tetrazolium test is to be used to find potential bladder carcinogens, it has to be tested on the bladder mucosa, and for lung carcinogens on lung tissue, etc.

Purchase *et al.* (1976), representing the staff of scientists at the Central Toxicology Laboratory of ICI Ltd., published a review paper in *Nature* with an evaluation of six short-term tests for detecting organic chemical carcinogens. The tetrazolium reduction test was listed as having a positive predictive value of only 40% for carcinogens, and a predictive value of 73% for non-carcinogens, giving a total accuracy of 57%; their conclusion was that this test performed poorly in all respects and was therefore of no general value.

However, there is a great difference between their use of the test and ours. We have only claimed that the tetrazolium test is *positive for skin carcinogens after topical application*, whereas Purchase *et al.* worked with a much more general definition, and they, for example, used the tetrazolium test on the skin to test for substances that are carcinogenic only for the liver or for the bladder. Here are some examples. (For references, see also *Survey of Compounds which have been tested for Carcinogenic Activity*, 1972–1973, Volume DHEW Publication (NIH) No. 75, Nat. Inst. of Health, Bethesda, 1977).

Benzidine was listed by Purchase *et al.* as negative according to the tetrazolium test, and positive on animal carcinogenicity. Hundreds of mice have been painted with benzidine, and only one papilloma, occurring in

1922, has been reported. Benzidine has never been shown to be a skin carcinogen following topical application. Benzidine is a urinary bladder carcinogen.

2-acetylaminofluoroene is listed as negative according to the tetrazolium test but positive for animal carcinogenicity. There is not a single report that shows that 2-acetylaminofluoroene is a skin carcinogen following topical application.

1-fluoro-2, 4-nitrobenzene has never been shown to be a complete skin carcinogen after direct application; tumours are elicited only in combination with DMBA or croton oil, or both.

Nitrosopholic acid has never been reported as being a skin carcinogen after painting. After injection into a large number of animals, four adenocarcinomas in the lung and no tumours on the skin were seen.

Quite recently we have done a blind test of *diethylstilboestrol*, which was positive in our test, and the two very similar substances trans-stilbene and oestradiol-17ß, which were both negative. This compares nicely with the carcinogenicity of diethylstilboestrol and the non-carcinogenicity of the two other substances. It should here be mentioned that diethylstrilboestrol has been repeatedly negative in the mutagenicity test of Ames.

The conclusion that the tetrazolium test for skin carcinogens is of no *general value* is thus self-evident, but this does not imply that it is of no value for skin carcinogenesis. On the contrary, my own experience of over a hundred substances, plus reports published by others, and even the detailed list of substances tested by the ICI Central Toxicology Laboratory, which they kindly have sent me as privileged information, show that, as a test for skin carcinogens, the tetrazolium method is as good a screening method as any of the other methods published, and it takes only 3–4 days to get a result.

The mechanism behind the increased deposition of formazan in tissues the first 1–3 days after exposure to a carcinogen is completely unexplained, and the test is empirical. However, Laerum (1969) has shown that there is a dissociation between oxygen consumption and formazan deposition the first few days after carcinogen application to the epidermis, and this points to cell injury with a block in the respiratory chain, and not to increased oxygen consumption. Detailed discussions of possible mechanisms can be found in Iversen (1962) and in Laerum (1969).

We are planning to try to elucidate the mechanism behind the tetrazolium test in greater detail if it turns out to work well on liver carcinogenesis.

Bibliography

Ben, M. and Valentini, J. E. (1965). Determination of potential carcinogenic materials by the Iversen and Evensen technique. *Proceedings of the Scientific Section of the Toilet Goods Association*, **43,** 44

Iversen, O. H. (1962). Effects of carcinogens on mitochondrial function. In O. H. Iversen and A. Evensen (eds.). *Experimental Skin Carcinogenesis in Mice, Acta Path. et Microbiol. Scand., Suppl.* **156,** 29

Iversen, O. H. and Devik, F. (1962). Effects of local roentgen irradiation on the rate of endogenous-dehydrogenase activity in the epidermis of hairless mice studied by means of a tetrazolium-reduction method. *Int. J. Radiat. Biol.*, **4,** 277

Iversen, O. H. (1963). An early test for possible skin carcinogens. *NCI Monograph*, **10,** 633

Iversen, O. H. and Laerum, O. D. (1964). The respiration of mouse epidermis after a single application of 3-methylcholanthrene in benzene. *Acta Path. Microbiol. Scand.*, **60,** 90

Iversen, O. H. (1963). An early test for possible skin carcinogens in the mouse: Effects of a benzacridine and of some tricycloquinazolines. *Nature (Lond.)*, **198,** 400

Iversen, O. H. (1961). An early test for possible skin carcinogens. *Nature (Lond.)*, **192,** 273

Iversen, O. H. (1962). An early test for possible skin carcinogens in the mouse: Effect of different doses of 3-methylcholanthrene in benzene solution. *Nature (Lond.)*, **196,** 181

Laerum, O. D. (1969). Studies of respiration and glycolysis of epidermal cells in relation to early skin carcinogenesis. Thesis. Norwegian University Press

Purchase, I. F. H., Longstaff, E., Ashby, J., Styles, J. A., Anderson, D., Lefevre, P. A. and Westwood, F. R. (1976). Evaluation of six short term tests for detecting organic chemical carcinogens and recommendations for their use. *Nature (Lond.)*, **264,** 624

Index

2-Acetamidofluorene, 39, 43
4-Acetamidofluorene, 34, 39, 41, 43, 44, 57
Acetylaminofluorene (AAF), metabolism of, 9, 68, 70, 122
Aflatoxins, 10, 22, 41, 43, 75, 114
Aldrin, 20
Alkylating agents, 65–67
  arizidines (ethyleneimines), 66
  as anticancer agents, 67
  bromohexitols, 66
  epoxides (oxiranes), 66
  nitrogen mustard, 66
  sulphonoxy alkenes (methane sulphonates), 66
Ames test, 30, 55–57, 122
  and diethylstilboestrol, 122
  reaction of agent with DNA in, 56
4-Aminoazobenzene, 34
2-Aminochrysene, 39, 44
6-Aminochrysene, 39, 44
Amylobarbitone, 47
Anthracene, 43
Arochlor 1254, 30, 33
Aromatic amines, 69
Arsenic, 114
Asbestos, 114

Bacterial test, 33, 56–58
  mutation, correct evaluation of, 57, 58
    incorrect evaluation of, 56
    sensitivity of, 58
Benefit of drugs, evaluation of, 110
Benz(a)anthracene, 43
Benz(a)pyrone, 40, 42, 46, 71
Benzidine, 20, 121
Bioassay, 91–101
  lifetime feeding protocols for, 91, 101
  mathematical model of, 91, 98
    breakdown of, 98
  thresholds of, 91
Biphenyl test, 45
Butylated N-hydroxyanisole, 73

Cancer testing and monitoring costs, 81–84
  break-even point, 82
  capital, 81
  capital investment, 82
  current legislative trends, 83
  tests, 81
  to industry, 83
Cancer principles, 21
Cantharidine, 120
Carcinomas, breast, in man and rodents, 7
  hepatocellular, in rats, 10
  liver, in man and rodent, 9
  lung, in man and rodent, 6
Carcinogenesis, by ultraviolet light, 90
  detection of, 20
  dose–response pattern, 90
  effect of diet on, 103
  factors influencing, 73
Carcinogenicity, biochemical mechanisms of, 65
  Mantel–Schneiderman model of, 92
  studies, in rodents, 89, 113
    predictive value of, 19, 20
  testing requirements, 106
    choice of compound, 107
    duration of test, 107
    method, 107
  tests, analysis of data from, 17
    animal, exactness of, 26
    dilemmas in, 6
    economics of, 79
    guidelines for, 19, 115
    object of, 23
    practical problems of large-scale experimentation, 28
    probability model of, 103
    protocols, validity and reproducibility of, 22
Carcinogens, definition of, 65, 77
  human, 113
  reaction with DNA, 31
  residues, measurement of binding to DNA, 35

Carcinogens, *cont.*
  species differences in susceptibility to, 29
  weak, 34
  see Electrophilic reactants
CDSM, *see* Regulatory authorities
Cell death, mechanism of, 67
Cell growth test, 39
Cell mutation test, 40, 46
Cell transformation test, 40, 46
Chlordane, 20
Chloroform, 65
Chromates, 114
Chromosomal binding and damage test, 35, 37, 46
Clones, *see* Tumours
Co-carcinogen, 22
COMA, *see* Regulatory authorities
CRM, *see* Regulatory authorities
CSM, *see* Regulatory authorities
CTC, *see* Regulatory authorities
Cut-off point, 62
Cycasin, 114
Cyclamate, 20
Cyclophosphamide, 39, 67
Cytogenetic analysis, 87

DDT, 20
DHSS, *see* Regulatory authorities
Dibutylnitrosamine, 43
Dieldrin, 20
Diethylstilboestrol, 36, 122
Dimethylaminoazobenzene, 43, 69
Dimethylbenz(a)anthracene, 43
Dimethylnitrosamine, 36, 39–41, 57
Disulfiram, 73
DNA, 31, 32, 35, 42, 56, 67
  damage to, 68
    measurement of, 75
  reaction with active metabolites, 31, 32
  reaction with carcinogens, 31, 32, 35
DNA repair test, 42, 43, 46
DOE, *see* Regulatory authorities
DPCP, *see* Regulatory authorities

Electrophilic reactants, 65–75
  biological properties of, 65
  factors influencing formation from precarcinogens, 73
  other ways of forming, 61
Endoplasmic reticulum, change in, 45, 46
Ethionine, 65
Ethoxycoumarin, 47
Ethyl carbamate (urethane), 36, 41, 71
Experimental design, statistical concepts of, 89

FACC, *see* Regulatory authorities

1-Fluoro-2, 4-nitrobenzene, 122

Gel electrophoresis, 45
Griseofulvin, 10
Guidelines for carcinogenicity studies in animals, *see* Carcinogenicity

Harman, 58
Heptachlor, 20
Heptacocarcinogens, 9
HSE, *see* Regulatory authorities

International Agency for Research on Cancer, 113

Liver cytochrome, 45
  drug-metabolizing enzymes in, 30
  lesions in mice, 10
  microsomes, 73
  S9 fraction, 56, 58
  see Carcinomas; Tetrazolium test; Tumours
Long-term tests for carcinogenicity, 1, 12, 23, 55, 57, 99
  animals for, 2
    autopsy and microscopy of, 4
    background incidence of disease in, 3
    diet of, 2
  general aspects of, 1
  procedures for, 3
    dose-levels, 3
    route of administration, 3
    test duration, 3
  statistical analysis of, 23, 24
    biological meaning of, 27
    Monte-Carlo study of, 99, 100
    significance, 23–25
  test compound in, 1

MAFF, *see* Regulatory authorities
Mantel–Schneiderman model, *see* Carcinogenicity
Maximum Tolerated Dose (MTD), 16
Medicines Act, 105, 117
Medicines Commission, *see* Regulatory authorities
Metabolites, active, formation of, 30
  nature of, 30
  reaction with DNA, 31
Methylazoxymethanol, 41
Methylcholanthrene (MCA), 30, 42, 44, 47, 120
11-Methylcyclopenta(a)phenanthrene, 41
2-Methyl 4-dimethylaminoazobenzene, 33, 39, 44
3′-Methyldimethylaminoazobenzene, 39, 44
Microbiological test, *see* Short-term tests

INDEX

NADPH, 30, 36, 45
ß-Naphthoflavone, 30, 46
ß-Naphthylamine, 20, 46
2-Naphthylamine, 34, 46
National Institute of Occupational Safety and Health, US, 113
4-Nitroquinoline-N-oxide, 39, 43
Nitrosophilic acid, 122
Nodules, liver, non-malignant, in man, 11, 12
  mammary, in progestogen-treated beagles, 8

Phenobarbitone, 11, 22, 30, 46
PL, *see* Regulatory authorities
Polycyclic hydrocarbons, 68
Potassium sorbate, 36
Precarcinogens, 65, 73
Preventive medicine, 29
Procarcinogens, 42, 43
Progestogens, testing requirements, 8, 107, 111
Proteins, abnormal, production and secretion of, 45

Quinoline, 36, 43

Radiolabelled tracers, decay rate of, 89
Regulatory authorities, 105–117
  Clinical Trial Certificate (CTC), 105, 106, 108, 109
  Committee on Dental and Surgical Materials (CDSM), 105
  Committee on Medical Aspects of Chemicals in Food, 105
  Committee on Review of Medicines (CRM), 105
  Committee on Safety of Medicines (CSM), 105, 106, 111, 117
  Consumer Products and the Environment (COMA), 114, 115
  Department of the Environment (DOE), 115
  Department of Health and Social Security (DHSS), 105, 111, 113, 114
    task and role of, 116
  Department of Prices and Consumer Protection (DPCP), 115
  Federal Drug Authority, 111
  Food Additives and Contaminants, (FACC), 115
  Ministry of Agriculture, Fisheries and Food (MAFF), 115
  Pesticides Safety Precaution Committee, 115
  Problems facing medicinal products, *see* Medicines Act
  Product Licences (PL), 105, 106, 108, 109
Response system, human, biological preparations to simulate, 32
  quality of, 34
Risk, assessment and minimization of, 20, 113
  evaluation of, 110
Risk–benefit analyses, 11, 109–111, 116
  assessment, decisions involving, 109
  problems of, 80
RNA, 67

Saccharin, 20, 36, 55
  sodium, 38
Sebaceous gland suppression test, 46
Selenium, 62
Short-term tests for carcinogenicity, 29, 33, 36, 42–46, 48, 55, 62, 75, 85, 115, 119
  criticism of, 62
  decision scheme for, 85, 86
  desirability of, 108, 109
  in vitro, 29
    ideal, 31
  microbiological, predictive value of, 55
  mutation, 103
  possible endpoints for, 32
  principles of, 30
  problems in assessing predictability of, 33
  range of concentrations, 62
  role of, 59
  scientific rationale for, 30
  types of, 35
  validation of, 34, 53
Sodium benzoate, 36
Statistical analysis, *see* Long-term tests for carcinogenicity
Sulphur mustard gas, 65, 75

TCCD, 46
Tetrazolium reduction test, 46, 119–122
  and bladder mucosa, 121
  and liver tissue, 120
  and lung tissue, 121
  basis for, 119
  possible mechanisms of, 122
Thiocetamide, 65
Tier one screening, 33, 47
  aim of, 48
  requirements of, 47
Tier two screening, 47
  uses of, 48
4-o-Tolylazo-o-toluidine, 36
Toxicity testing, effort and cost of, 87
Triphenyltetrazolium chloride, 119
Tumours, background incidence of, 103
  breast, 7
  cells, clones of, 98

Tumours, *cont.*
comparison of, in animals and man, 17
development of, cell mutation as primary cause, 32
growth, inhibition of, 39
induced and spontaneous, in animals, 17
liver, 8
lung, 5
phases of induction by chemicals, 31
pulmonary, due to cigarette smoking, 79
qualitative appraisal of, in tests for, 12

Urea, 36

Vinyl carbamate, 71